# notes

from a naturopath

# notes

## from a naturopath

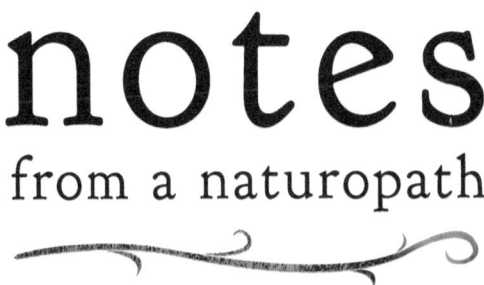

Thomasina G. Copenhaver RN, BSN, ND

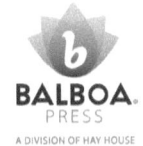

BALBOA.
PRESS

A DIVISION OF HAY HOUSE

Permission granted to include the chapter, "Juicing with Jay Kordich—The "Juiceman" answers from Jay Kordich. Jay wrote it and it can be found here and on my blog.

Balboa Press books may be ordered through booksellers or by contacting:

Balboa Press
A Division of Hay House
1663 Liberty Drive
Bloomington, IN 47403
www.balboapress.com
1 (877) 407-4847

Because of the dynamic nature of the Internet, any web addresses or links contained in this book may have changed since publication and may no longer be valid. The views expressed in this work are solely those of the author and do not necessarily reflect the views of the publisher, and the publisher hereby disclaims any responsibility for them.

The author of this book does not dispense medical advice or prescribe the use of any technique as a form of treatment for physical, emotional, or medical problems without the advice of a physician, either directly or indirectly. The intent of the author is only to offer information of a general nature to help you in your quest for emotional and spiritual well-being. In the event you use any of the information in this book for yourself, which is your constitutional right, the author and the publisher assume no responsibility for your actions.

Any people depicted in stock imagery provided by Thinkstock are models, and such images are being used for illustrative purposes only. Certain stock imagery © Thinkstock.

Printed in the United States of America.

ISBN: 978-1-4525-2177-0 (sc)
ISBN: 978-1-4525-2178-7 (hc)
ISBN: 978-1-4525-2176-3 (e)

Library of Congress Control Number: 2014915988

Balboa Press rev. date: 10/20/2014

# Contents

# A Note from the Author

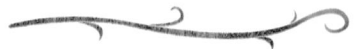

Everything you hope to accomplish in this lifetime is dependent upon your understanding of how your body works at the cellular level. Every one of us has the innate, God-given ability to heal. You are a miracle—your body is preprogrammed to think for itself, and it knows perfectly and exactly how to restore itself to balance. But you need an owner's manual to understand how this works. The problem is that most people try to eliminate *symptoms*, and when that is accomplished, believe they are healed, and then continue to engage in the behavior that *caused* the symptoms to begin with.

Taking a pill for a symptom without treating the underlying cause is like taking the batteries out of a smoke detector to stop the annoying alarm while the house burns down.

*Notes from a Naturopath* is like your personal GPS system. This book puts you in the driver's seat, and you determine where you want to go. You decide your personal definition of health and how you want to get there. You decide your truth. Some people are sick and tired of feeling sick and tired—and want the fastest way to health. Others take a cautious approach and make changes slowly, with grace. I am not talking about substituting an herb for a pill; I am talking about developing lasting *lifestyle changes*. Most lasting changes take place slowly, one by one, over time. This means becoming conscious of what we put in our bodies, what we allow past the door to our minds, and the personal choices we make every day that determine our health.

This book is designed to be a beginning. It takes you from where you are right now and gives you the wisdom of the ancients, the cutting-edge science that supports that wisdom, and the links and resources to decide your own truth. The best research is that which is carried out personally by having an open mind, open eyes, and open ears.

What could be more empowering than taking control of your health? At a time when health care and insurance options are so confusing and stressful, taking responsibility for your own health is calming and reassuring. All healing has a place. The technology offered by Western medicine and the ancient techniques of naturopathic doctors are finally combined in one easy-to-understand "owner's manual." This uniquely organized book clearly explains, in simple terms, our body's innate ability to heal.

My role as a naturopath is *not* to diagnose or prescribe—nor is it to advise one treatment or philosophy versus another. Everyone is at different stages of consciousness. My intent is to awaken, educate, empower, and inspire you to make your own personal choices based on knowledge, as opposed to fear. The health I am talking about is vital, energetic health and not just the absence of disease. Each of us must choose our own path. My intent is to speak my truth, based on my experiences—not to convince you but to empower you.

Namaste.

# "What did the Author mean" —Resources versus Bibliography

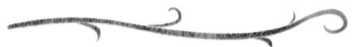

I learned the hard way that the only person who *really* knows what the author means is the author.

In writing and researching this book, I chose to put "Resources" at the end of each chapter as opposed to using footnotes or one long Bibliography at the end. When I read a book, I find footnotes distracting. I want to stop reading and go find the article or product mentioned! The first three chapters of my book set the stage for my basic philosophy. The chapters that follow are unique and individual, and could be read alone. For example, you may be interested in the story of my husband's experience with cancer, or natural approaches to Lyme Disease. At the end of each of those chapters you will find the articles, books, products, and videos that I used to research and write that chapter. If you want to explore the individual subject, or watch a video, or look up a product that I use and recommend, you don't have to search through hundreds of references. It is listed at the end of the chapter in which it is mentioned.

I state this over and over in the book, but I feel it is important to understand, "What did the author mean" from the start; that the material presented here represents my truth based upon my thirty years of research and experience, and it is my intention that it will empower you to find your truth. The resources I use are personally selected and trusted to the best of my ability. I am not affiliated with any company and do not receive any royalties or compensation for recommending any person or product.

In the E-Book version, the Resources are directly linked in the chapters by clicking on the corresponding link in the text. However, it is my sincere hope that this book reaches all those who seek the information within it, regardless of Internet accessibility. I personally love physical, hard/soft cover books. So I have gone back and tried to put as much information about how to find the resources listed, as possible. Many of the books and products are only available online, so some computer access is necessary. All resources listed can also be found on my website: www. notesfromanaturopath.com in the "Resources" section, and on the corresponding blog post.

Please keep in mind that websites get updated, new information becomes available, and links sometime become inactive. I have updated every link and added all new information or the most recent books as of this final edit.

# Acknowledgments

Thanks to God for listening to my endless query—"Is this really what I am supposed to do?"

Thanks to my family for all their support.

Thank you to Dr. Robert O. Young for his research, caring, and "New Biology"

Thank you to Jay Kordich for teaching me everything I know and understand about juicing.

Thank you to David Wolfe for his amazing research on Longevity and Nutrition; for his conferences, videos, products, and events that bring together true experts in the fields of health, longevity and epigenetics. I have learned so much and I am grateful.

Thanks to Truth Calkins and Donna Schwenk for helping me understand the role of bacteria in the cycle of life.

Thanks to Noah Urban and mazuzu.com for the tireless work on the cover design.

Thanks to Gail Seib for checking my work and being so supportive.

Thanks to Rev. Lawrence J. Gesy, M.Div.M.S.—author of the book, *The Hem of His Garment* (available on Amazon.com) for his faith in me. You inspire me. I adore you.

Thanks to my friends who have supported and believed in me. I appreciate you more than words can say.

chapter one

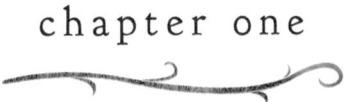

# Frame Each Day with "Vitamin G": Gratitude

*What is wrong is always available, but so is what's great.*
—Anthony Robbins

Gratitude is everything. How many people do you know who have everything—and are always miserable? Why is it that people who have so little always seem to be happy? Gratitude; it does a body good (to paraphrase that milk commercial from the eighties).

I learned a lot about gratitude from being a nurse. I learned the value of being able to swat away annoying flies from patients who couldn't. Have you ever thought about that? I'll bet not. You might think about it the next time a mosquito lands on you. When you see someone confined to bed, unable to move any part of his body, except perhaps to blink, unable to speak or swallow so he is fed through a feeding tube surgically inserted into his stomach, unable to bend his arms or legs to get the least bit comfortable, essentially stiff from the neck down, beads of sweat on his face, the daily intractable pain reflected in his eyes—and you understand that while you go home day after day, this is his life. A fly lands on his eyelids or nose and starts walking around. You appreciate the ability to swat away a fly.

That someone was the uncle who raised me. A man who fought in three wars and was afraid of nothing had a spinal cord stroke ten days after I gave birth to my first son—twenty-four hours after I moved halfway across the country. Most of us spend so much time complaining about all the things our bodies *can't* do that we often fail to appreciate the miraculous things our bodies can do.

Cancer patients taught me gratitude as well. There I was complaining about having to go pick up my kids, or driving in traffic, and I would think of my thirty-five-year-old niece who was enduring God-awful cancer treatments for the *privilege* of having one more minute, one more day—to do the same.

In his program *Get the Edge* (see end of chapter for details), Tony Robbins talks about "The Hour of Power." First thing in the morning you move, breathe, and think about everything for which you are grateful. Movement like walking, deep breathing, and engaging your body and your emotions together—being grateful for the people, the moments, the experiences that bring you joy. Tony says, "Movement is energy" and "emotion comes from motion."

I like to call it framing your day with gratitude. My son laughs at me because I take pictures of things every day to "appreciate" them. If one tiny flower blooms in the driveway, I take a picture and appreciate that it bloomed all by itself. I am grateful for sunrises and moonbeams. I love morning glories and plant them every year to remind me of my mother who died when I was eight. She loved morning glories and roses, which she grew under jars.

Tony says life is all about magic *"moments"*—not just big days or special events like birthdays. Be grateful for these moments each day—and capture them in a journal—or write them on a piece of paper and put them in a jar. What made you smile or laugh? Did you see a breathtaking sunset and go, *"Wow!"* Review these accumulated moments weekly or monthly. And at the end of the year, take them out and reflect on how many great moments you have had every day. And every day becomes an extraordinary life.

You need to be grateful in order to love yourself. You can't love yourself if you don't love your body. Your body loves you—all the time. Your body takes such good care of you that oftentimes you take for granted just how much your body does, until it breaks down. Gratitude is the antidote to *stress*. When you are grateful and happy, you secrete happy hormones. Your blood and saliva become more alkaline, and as you move and breathe, your tissues become oxygenated. By some accounts, exercise alone can cut your risk of cancer by 50 percent and eliminate depression—without side effects.

Elevate your mood even further and add some music and Tony's favorite positive mantra, "Every day in every way, I'm _____." Twelve years ago, that mantra for my husband was, "Every day in every way, I'm beating this, I'm cancer free." My defensive lineman, high school football playing husband was not one to walk around chanting affirmations first thing in the morning (or any other time), nor was he used to carrying around a pocket Angel to anchor those words throughout the day. But you must frame your day and continue to affirm and anchor thoughts of gratitude, as opposed to those of fear. It worked! He is cancer free, still. Try to spend the first hour—or thirty minutes, fifteen minimum—of your day this way.

How many reasons do you have to love your body and self? Prepare to be amazed. When I first read this information from my mentor and friend Dr. Robert Young, I was truly surprised. I never really thought about it. All the following calculations are courtesy of Dr. Young and I am very grateful because science is my passion—*math is* not. You will hear lots more about Dr. Young in many chapters that follow.

According to Dr. Young, "At maturity, the human skeleton contains about 165 bones, delicately and perfectly adjusted. There are approximately 500 muscles. The heart is 6 inches in length and 4 inches in diameter and beats 70 times per minute, 4200 times per hour, 100,800 per day, and 36,720,000 per year. At each beat, two and one-half ounces of blood are thrown out of it, 175 ounces per minute, 656 pounds per hour, or about 8 tons a day."

Now you get the math thing ...

Dr. Young continues: "All the blood in the body passes through the heart every three minutes. And during 70 years it lifts 270,000,000 tons of blood.

"The lungs contain about a gallon of air at their usual degree of inflation. We breathe, on average, 1200 breaths per hour and inhale 600 gallons of air, or 24,000 gallons daily. The aggregate surface of air cells of the lungs exceed 20,000 square inches, an area nearly equal to that of a room 12 feet square.

"The average weight of the brain of an adult is three pounds, eight ounces. The average female brain is 2 pounds, 4 ounces. The convolutions of a woman's brain cells and tissues are finer and more delicate in fiber and mechanism, which accounts for our intuition.

"The nerves are all connected with the brain directly, or by the spinal marrow, but nerves receive their nutrition from the blood, and their motive power from the solar plexus dynamic. These nerves, together with their branches and minute ramifications, probably exceed ten million in number.

"The skin is composed of three layers and varies from one-eighth to one-quarter of an inch in thickness. The average area of skin is estimated to be about 2,000 square inches. Atmospheric pressure, being 14 pounds per square inch, subjects a person of medium size to a pressure of 40,000 pounds. Each square inch of skin contains 3,500 sweat tubes or perspiratory pores (which may be likened to drain tiles) one-fourth of an inch in length, making an aggregate length of the entire surface of the body 201,166 feet, or a tube for draining the body nearly 40 miles in length.

"We take in an average of five and a half pounds of food and drink each day, which amounts to one ton of solid and liquid nutrition annually. In seventy years, we eat and drink one thousand times our body weight."

Thank you, Dr. Young, for all those calculations!

This is just the beginning of understanding how your body works at the cellular level. Your body *loves* you. Your body knows perfectly and exactly how to heal itself. My role is to educate, awaken, empower, and inspire you to understand healing at the cellular level, and to achieve radiant health—not just the absence of disease—but feel great energy to fulfill what it is that you came to this planet to accomplish.

Are you grateful? Are you ready? Follow me ...


## RESOURCES:

*Get The Edge* CD set from 2000 by Anthony Robbins: Day 1—**Your Hour of Power.** http://www.tonyrobbins.com/

Young, Robert O., and Shelley Redford Young. *Sick and tired?: reclaim your inner terrain.* Pleasant Grove, UT: Woodland Pub., 2001.

www.phmiracleliving.com. (This is Dr. Young's website if you want to search for products, his articles of health blog, or any further information)

## chapter two

Fuel for the Journey—
You Can't Buy Energy in a Can

It has been scientifically proven that electromagnetic fields exist around every living being. Each of us has an energy signature or essence.

Flowers take nutrients from the soil and absorb them through their roots. As they grow, they are energized and animated by sunlight and rain. A seed becomes a flower. A rose becomes a rose. When you think of a rose, or smell a rose, that flower transfers its energy to you. Florists, poets, and perfume makers all use the essence of a rose to appeal to your senses. When you give a rose to a loved one, it lifts their Spirit, and they feel good.

And so it is with plants. Plants take their individual nutrient requirements from the soil. A tomato seed takes elements like nitrogen and calcium, opens its leaves to absorb and store the energy of the sun; quenches its thirst with rain, and becomes a ripe juicy tomato. A tomato plant has a different energy signature than a carrot or a red pepper, even though they all share the same garden soil. When you eat a carrot, it transfers a different energy signature than a pepper or tomato. A carrot does not look, smell or taste like anything other than a carrot. Gardeners rotate plants so that the soil doesn't become depleted of any one nutrient. Green plants give you their rich green chlorophyll, which is identical to human blood except for the center atom of magnesium; in a red blood cell the center atom is iron. When you eat green leafy vegetables or drink the juice of wheatgrass, they enliven and energize you by *building* healthy red blood cells in your small intestine.

Healing your body at the cellular level is all about energy. Energy cannot be created nor destroyed—it can only be transformed.

We are all miraculous, light filled beings. We are electromagnetic. Every thought, every heartbeat, sends electrical signals that power your body. Nerve impulses (signals) are electrical "pulses" that receive information externally and internally, interpret that data, and instantly communicate it. Every cell in your body possesses infinite intelligence to interpret and act upon that information to maintain balance and harmony. Therefore, every cell in your body must be energized with electrical power— makes sense—right?

What powers us, at the individual cellular level, is a miraculous biochemical balance of minerals, salts, oxygen and pure water. Take away any of these critical elements, and the human body would dry up, stop breathing, and die. Therefore, the fuel to energize and power our bodies *must* contain all those natural elements. Our fuel comes from the air we breathe, the food we eat, the water we drink, and the thoughts we communicate. Yes ... thoughts are electromagnetic. Specifically, natural salt from the earth increases the electrical potential of water and conducts electricity. All the fluids of the human body are salted; blood, saliva, tears, sweat, and urine. You are the salt of the earth for real!

Our entire nervous system pulses with magnetic currents. Wherever there is a flow of electrical current, there is also magnetism because the two must always go together. Wherever you have a transmission, you also have a reception. Wherever there is electricity flowing, it both attracts other currents and also transmits them. An electric motor does the same—there are two magnets with a copper coil in between—the coil captures the energy between the magnets. The electrical power of the human body controls every function it must carry out--from the rhythm of your heartbeat to the amount of blood flowing through your capillaries, to your light and dark reception, or circadian rhythm.

The cell structure of the human body is the same. You have a nucleus and you have cytoplasm. The nucleus is the positive pole and the cytoplasm the negative. You have conductive minerals (sodium, potassium, magnesium, calcium, etc.), and you have fluid (water) that is contained by an outer cell membrane made of lipids (fat). Every cell membrane is made of lipids—a reason why you *need* cholesterol. Coenzyme Q10 is made in your liver from cholesterol. CoQ10 is critical for mitochondrial respiration. Statin drugs block the production of Coenzyme Q10.

Inside each cell are the mitochondria. The mitochondria are the power stations. By the process of aerobic (with oxygen) respiration, the mitochondria convert oxygen and nutrients into ATP (adenosine triphosphate). ATP is your electrical currency of life, or life force. If your heart stops beating, a defibrillator can deliver an electrical shock to attempt to restore heart rhythm. If you are struck by lightning, the uncontrolled electrical shock can kill you. The mitochondria of the cells are also responsible for telling the cells when it is time to die so they can be replaced by new cells.

Built into the infinite intelligence of every cell is a process called *"apoptosis."* When your body determines that a cell is no longer useful, enzymes called *capases* break apart and destroy the DNA, shrink the nucleus and cytoplasm, and shut down the mitochondria. (Stay away from that stuff!) The cell membrane remains intact, but the cell quickly shrinks from surrounding cells and dies without the power of the mitochondria and the brain of the nucleus. These cells are then eliminated. This is a *natural process*. This is your body getting rid of old, tired cells to make room for new, healthy ones. This process also occurs in a developing baby—the tissue between your fingers and toes (the webbing) is unnecessary, so your body removes it from the fetus. And you have ten individual fingers. And ten toes. Amazing!

The process of apoptosis is, according to cutting-edge cancer research, where cancer begins.

The primary cause of cancer, from an energetic perspective, is mitochondrial failure. Cutting edge research supports this, but Dr. Otto Warburg won a Nobel prize for his discovery back in the 1920s that cancer cells get their energy by consuming huge amounts of glucose and breathing without oxygen (anaerobic respiration). Dr. Warburg hypothesized that the mitochondria of cancer cells must be different or damaged, because normal healthy cells are powered by aerobic (oxygen) respiration.

Ancient man ate locally and seasonally. He did not count calories (units of energy) or read labels. He did not worry about whether his grains were gluten free or if eating too much coconut meat would make his thighs look big. He did not depend on a newscaster or TV doctor to tell him what to eat. All his food was "organic" because there were no pesticides or man made adulterated "genetically modified" foods. Ancient man had instinct and intellect. He foraged for food or grew his own food. Food gave him the energy he needed to survive. By some estimates, ancient man could run 28 miles per hour from predators. How fast can you run? In fact, the Tarahumara of Mexico could run for days with only freshly picked Chia Seed in their cheeks or in a drink with water. Chia seeds give you omega oils, fiber, and lasting energy. In his book, *Born To Run*, author Christopher McDougall refers to the Tarahumara Chia drink known as *iskiate,* as "ten thousand year old Red Bull." Ancient man didn't read the book—he knew it instinctively and intellectually because his ancestors experienced it and passed along that information from generation to generation.

When you eat blueberries, they transfer their energy signature to you. Natural, live, fresh foods are "anabolic," meaning they build up red blood cells. They have their own enzymes, minerals, and properties that do not take energy from you. They give up their life force so that you may have vital life force.

Let's say you would rather eat your blueberries in a pie. Cooking your blueberries over 110 degrees destroys the enzymes and vitamins. Blueberry pie is "catabolic" which means, "that which tears down." When you eat cooked food you still build red blood cells, but they lack vital energy because the heating of the blueberries destroys their energy signature. The tissues built from cooked or highly processed canned or packaged food lacks live enzymes and has no nutrient value. If your inner terrain is built from only catabolic food, you expend more energy than you build up and cells begin to self-destruct (apoptosis) because their environment is toxic and acidic. Innate intelligence determines these energy deficient cells to be useless and sends those capases to internally implode them. The human body does not run on carbohydrates, it runs on energy transferred from natural enzyme and nutrient rich fuel.

Your body must have a certain pH level in order to maintain the electrical current that powers your heart, brain, and nerve receptors. The pH scale goes from 0 (being pure acid that kills you instantly) to 14 (pure alkaline). You must maintain a blood pH of 7.36 (slightly alkaline) for the blood to effectively carry oxygen and nutrients to the cells and remove waste. An acid pH strips red blood cells of their electrical charge. Think of an alkaline battery. An alkaline battery is stored electrical *potential*. When batteries go dead, they have lost their electrical potential. Your body needs electrical potential in the form of stored energy to neutralize acid. Green plants transfer their stored energy and light (chlorophyll) to you when you eat them. Cheeseburgers do not.

Fuel for the journey through life must be mostly natural, live, raw, organic fruits, vegetables, and natural unadulterated grains, seeds, and nuts that transfer their energy to you. Notice this does NOT include any diet or label like "gluten free," "fat free," "raw," "meat free," etc. Those are man made labels and have nothing to do with life force energy. When you are filled with life force energy, you transfer your life force to those around you. You can't wait to get up every day, you are filled with gratitude for another sunrise, for the present moment, you see the beauty and the lesson in everything, your eyes shine, your skin is moist and glowing, and you smile a lot. You feel so amazingly alive that you can't help but share the feeling. You radiate **love**. How many middle aged humans do you know that fit into that category? The highest life force or essence of a human being is love.

Is this fuel "fast" or always "convenient?" Not without planning, preparation and possibly a juicer. Neither is cancer treatment, hauling around an oxygen tank, or packing a motorized cart along with your bikini and a case filled with all your pills when you hit the beach. The good news is—you get to choose! Every minute of every day you can choose to be grateful, to consciously select what you put into your body, and to nourish your Soul. Or you can be sick, tired, and clueless.

Let's take it one step further. Suppose you made the blueberry pie yesterday and your sweet old uncle drops by today for a visit. Yes, he would love some warm blueberry pie—don't go to any trouble—just pop it in the microwave for a minute ...

Now you have moved from a fresh blueberry that was filled with sweet nourishment to build healthy red blood cells-- to beyond catabolic and entering free radical, possible cancer causing territory. You have now internally exploded and radiated the blueberry. Structurally, energetically, and chemically it is no longer a blueberry.

Microwave cooking or even reheating, DE-natures and deteriorates cells. Cells are broken apart—neutralizing their electrical potential. This violates natural law. This destroys their energy signature. And keep in mind—we are talking about real food that actually had electron potential. Microwaving anything from a plastic package "foraged" from a vending machine had no electron potential to begin with. In fact, ancient man would not even recognize it as "food."

Cells subjected to this form of electromagnetic radiation are forcefully made to reverse polarity. No atom or molecule known to man can withstand the violent friction of being imploded internally or DE-formed (also known as structural isomerism). Free radicals are created by the collateral damage. They are positive ions searching for electrons. They deplete your healthy cells of their negative electrons, leaving them damaged.

You have now transformed your inner terrain into a state of energy emergency. This means that instead of normal mitochondrial aerobic respiration, these deformed cells switch to anaerobic respiration and begin to ferment. If you only eat food that is cooked over 110 degrees, is processed, gluten or fat free, artificially sweetened, filled with pesticides, and/or microwaved— over time—significant DE-generative changes will occur in your blood. Your energy/electron-deprived red blood cells will become lifeless and anemic from lack of iron. Simply by adding fresh organic fruits and vegetables from a local farmer's market or grown in your front yard, patio, or garden—can put the life force back in your blood. One simple thing—like growing wheatgrass and juicing it, or trying a green drink or smoothie, or adding a salad made fresh from your garden—one simple thing can make a huge difference in whether you build healthy, beautiful, oxygen rich red blood cells, or sick and tired ones.

Jay Kordich, a.k.a. "The Juiceman," taught me everything I know about juicing. He is so knowledgeable and shares his passion for the power of fresh juice in healing the body, freely and with great love. Jay is a cancer survivor. He wrote a chapter for me on juicing versus blending.

Nature draws us to plants by our senses. Natural foods enrich, strengthen, energize and heal your body at the cellular level by offering you their stored energy and light. When you consume them, you too become a vibrant, electromagnetic, light-filled being. The ancients called that light "shen," or "spirit" ("that which can not be named") and use an analogy of a candle. The flame of the candle burns energy—but the purpose of the candle is the *light.*

You are the salt of the earth. You are the light of the world. Shine on ...

## RESOURCES:

Studies about cancer and mitochondrial function:
M.Yu, "Somatic Mitochondrial DNA Mutations in Human Cancers," Advances in Clinical Chemistry 57 (2012):99-138

The body electric explained with excellent video about the elements:
http://articles.mercola.com/sites/articles/archive/2014/03/01/body-electricity-grounding.aspx?x_cid=20140731_healthtip_facebookdoc

Excellent articles about Statin drugs and mitochondrial dysfunction
http://www.ncbi.nlm.nih.gov/pmc/articles/PMC3096178/

http://www.drsinatra.com/coq10-facts-what-you-should-know

http://articles.mercola.com/sites/articles/archive/2011/02/12/dr-duane-graveline-on-cholesterol-and-coq10.aspx

Article about Microwave lawsuits and follow up studies:
http://www.mercola.com/article/microwave/hazards2.htm

http://www.menshealth.com.sg/mh-runners/secrets-tarahumara-runners

http://www.chrismcdougall.com/blog/2010/09/10000-year-old-red-bull/

Jay Kordich—For all things juice related, I send you to Jay's website for a wealth of information and resources. Jay wrote the juicing chapter and graciously allowed me to share it on my personal blog, and in this book. www.jaykordich.com

chapter three

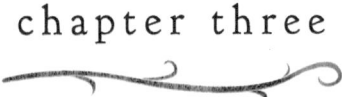

# There Is Only One Disease

*If the fish is sick, change the water.*
—Dr. Robert Young

So much of our lives are shaped by our lifestyle choices. Do you consciously decide each day to honor your body—the temple of your soul? Do you consciously think about what you can do to live a life that is filled with energy and vibrant health so you can fulfill your purpose? Do you come with an owner's manual?

Remember, at the cellular level we are electromagnetic beings. Our bodies function by sending pulses of electricity. This is carried out by the nervous system, which communicates these signals from the brain throughout the body. If you have ever heard of an ECG (electrocardiogram of the heart) or an EEG (electroencephalogram of the brain) or if you love the TV show *House* like I do, you know these are tests to measure electrical activity. This electrical activity is translated into line tracings on paper or computer screen. Disruptions in the electrical pulses are not treated by administering energy drinks, coffee, soda, pork rinds, gummy bears, or cheese fries. If you are headed toward a flat line, an IV is inserted into your vein to give you fluid and minerals like sodium and potassium.

These keep you alive. Polluting your bloodstream with junk food that is devoid of any real nutrition causes a buildup of acid. *Acid is the cause of all disease.*

Acid pollution is everywhere. Anything that emits positive ions (units of energy) is not good for the human body. We must have negative ions to survive. Let's start with the air we breathe.

At one time the magnetic force in the universe was 4.0 gauss. Now it is 0.4 gauss. Inside your house is 0 gauss. Negative ions are being stripped out of our world by electromagnetic pollution. Highly charged electrical fields with 600-plus watt power lines is an example of this. We are exposed to all sorts of electrical devices such as cell phones and computers. This type of pollution creates positive ions and changes our cell structure. One of the biggest lobbies in Washington DC is for the protection of electronic devices. In order to get the highest concentration of *negative ions*, you would need to stand by a waterfall, climb to the top of a mountain, walk along the beach, or take a romantic walk after a spring rain. That wonderful *feeling* you get from being in those places comes from negative ions that also change your cell structure—but in a positive way.

You also create acid by what you think, eat, and drink. Whatever you think about becomes what you emotionalize or how you feel. That emotion creates a magnetic field. Every so-called "disease" that manifests on the outside was first created and magnetized by a thought on the inside. *Stressful* thoughts turn everything to acid—from saliva, to excess stomach acid, to diarrhea. Stress is another word for thoughts of fear, anger, and frustration.

When you eat foods that are cooked at high temperatures, you destroy the enzymes. Enzymes are the life force of food. Remember, live foods are the only foods that transfer their solar energy directly to our red blood cells. Dr. Paul Kouchakoff showed (back in 1930) that eating a diet that was more than 51 percent cooked food caused your body to react to that food the same as if a virus or bacteria were invading it, causing your immune system to react to a false alarm. Cooking oils begin to oxidize at high temps and break down, creating free-radical damage to the food. Free radicals are harmful particles that are sometimes generated by excessive intake of poor nutrition, physical or emotional stress, environmental pollution, toxin exposure, surgery, toxic metals and radiation. Free radicals have a free electron that disrupts the integrity of cell membranes. Because they are so destructive, cells have innate defenses that neutralize them. Molecules called antioxidants neutralize them; which include vitamins, minerals, and special chemicals secreted called thiols (two of which are glutathione and alpha-lipoic acid). All processed food is pure junk.

Remember, your body loves you and is always working to bring you into balance. Your body is preprogrammed to miraculously think for itself. Every cell possesses infinite intelligence and communication. Everything you need—to live with vibrant energy and to accomplish your purpose in this lifetime—is dependent upon your understanding of how your body works at the cellular level.

We have lost our connection to nature. We must follow the laws of nature. Basic principles of naturopathy are restful sleep, clean air, sunshine, clean water, and fresh fruits and vegetables. This is how the ancients lived. Today, man lives indoors, in artificial light, tethered to a cell phone while staring at a computer, sitting for hours and eating food that is completely devoid of any nutrients. You can't break the law forever. If you follow the laws of nature, you will have a strong immune system and healthy inner terrain.

If your bloodstream is polluted with toxins, your elimination systems of respiration, perspiration, urination, and defecation back up. If your body can't eliminate acidic wastes, it must still remove them from your bloodstream to keep them away from your vital organs or you will die. So your body stores toxins in fat deposits. If you are one of those people who are lean and muscular, the acids have nowhere to go. This is why you sometimes hear about a runner who is lean and appears healthy but drops dead of a heart attack. Excessive exercise also causes lactic tissue acidosis. A little fat is not a bad thing. Fat is protective, as you will see later.

You must maintain the *alkalinity* of the blood. You must become your own inner terrain scientist. So many young people take pill after pill in an attempt to get their body back into balance—but in our modern Western medical model of health, these things are unnatural and foreign to the true process of healing. Without alkaline reserves to buffer acid, your immune system will become overwhelmed—your T-cells and "natural killer cells" (white blood cells that defend you and provide immunity) will decrease, your bone marrow dries up, and you won't produce strong, oxygen-rich red blood cells. When surrounded by an environment low in oxygen and high in acid, healthy cells decrease and opportunistic bacteria (like candida) seize the opportunity to take over. As your pH level changes and drops below 7.3 due to the lack of alkaline foods and drinks, you acquire more packed acids and toxins—the environment becomes more acidic and hospitable for these bacteria to grow stronger—and eventually they overtake you, the host. Bacteria do their job very well. They break down decaying matter and return it to the earth. If your body lacks vital energy and your diet lacks vital nutrients and is filled with sugar and processed carbohydrates, and your thoughts and emotions are negative, then bacteria go from facilitating vital functions like making the B Vitamins, Vitamin K, producing serotonin and sending out white blood cells--to breaking down toxins and returning them to the earth from your organs of elimination. You must maintain beneficial good bacteria by eating live fruits and vegetables and fermented foods. When good bacteria grow and colonize in your gut, bad bacteria lose their territory and are eliminated. With bacteria, it is always a matter of numbers. Antibiotics kill bacteria. They do not replenish them. Bacteria are your immune system. Every diagnosis by a medical doctor can be traced to an underlying root cause of acidity that threw your *inner terrain into disequilibrium.*

I had never heard of the importance of "pH balance" until I purchased the *Get the Edge* program by Anthony Robbins on New Year's Eve 1999. There I was at midnight, sitting all alone, flipping through channels, having my own little pity party—the singer Prince told me I should be partying—it *was*, after all, 1999.

But everyone was asleep and I was exhausted. I was coming off three really difficult months. My second son's birth in September had been difficult—my epidural failed, I felt every stitch as they sewed me up, I almost bled to death, and my son inhaled blood and was whisked away to neonatal ICU moments after being born.

He spent fourteen days there, during which time his lung collapsed and he was put on a ventilator. One of the saddest days of my life was leaving the hospital without him. When he did come home, he cried continuously. For the first time in my life, I asked my doctor for antidepressants.

He refused. "I've known you since you were sixteen—you're not depressed. You just need some quality sleep. I'll pay for a hotel room for you—let your husband watch your baby—but you don't need antidepressants."

So when I turned on the QVC channel and saw Anthony Robbins (I already had an older program and his book) and listened to him for an hour (he is so inspiring), I bought the program because I needed to feel grateful for my life and my blessings again. I needed energy and vitality and a new lease on life.

Little did I know of the challenges waiting for me right around the corner. Even though I chose to be a stay-at-home mom for my boys, I was about to put all my nursing skills to the test with my oldest son breaking the bone in his arm completely in two, right above his elbow—requiring surgery and months of therapy for a nerve palsy—my husband being diagnosed with cancer, and my return to graduate school at age forty-six to become a naturopathic doctor.

I put *Get the Edge* on my bookshelf for many months before I even opened it. I will be forever grateful to Anthony Robbins for the wealth of information contained on those CDs, which changed my life.

## RESOURCES:

Robbins, Anthony. *Get the Edge* audio CD, 2000.

This was my original book on pH Balance:
Young R., Shelley Redford Young. *Sick and Tired?: Reclaim Your Inner Terrain*, Pleasant Grove, UT: Woodland Publishing, 2000.

Great article explaining negative ions:
http://www.webmd.com/balance/features/negative-ions-create-positive-vibes.

This article explains inflammation from eating cooked food:
http://www.healthbeyondhype.com/leukocytosis-toxic-reactions-to-eating-highly-heated-food-ezp-135.html.

Information from Dr. Young's website:
http://www.phmiracleliving.com/t-faq-science-of-ph.aspx.

http://articlesofhealth.blogspot.com/2013/10/acidity-and-alkalinity-can-change-cell.html.

This article lists 233 published papers on the "Efficacy of a Plant-Based Alkaline Nutrient-Rich pH Miracle Diet in the Treatment of Cancer."
http://articlesofhealth.blogspot.com/2014/02/233-published-papers-on-efficacy-of.html

# Cholesterol, Diabetes, and Alzheimer's—Understanding the Dangers of Statin Drugs

All of the above have something in common with a Ferrari. The final *Jeopardy!* answer is: "What is 'good oil?'"

If you were to ask the owner of a beautiful Ferrari what kind of oil he or she puts in the car to keep it running in peak performance, he or she would more than likely be able to tell you. In fact, if someone owns a beautiful, Italian-made, top-of-the-line car, that owner has probably read the owner's manual cover to cover. In fact, he or she could more than likely tell you everything there was to know about the car and offer to take you for a ride to show it off. The owner probably uses only the highest-quality fuel and the purest-quality oil, and makes sure the radiator is filled with water and antifreeze and the battery is free of corrosion.

If you were to ask that same car owner what kind of oil he or she puts into his or her body to keep it running in peak performance, that car owner would probably be clueless. Would he or she even know why good oil was needed? If there was a part of the body that functioned like a battery and could be "recharged," would this person know where to find it? How to recharge it? I'd say there were probably two chances: slim and none.

Just like a fine, exquisitely made sports car, your body needs high-quality oil to keep it lubricated. *Your liver, that miraculous detoxifier and filter, produces cholesterol because it is essential to every single cell in your body, and crucial to protecting you from acids that can destroy you.*

Cholesterol has many *crucial* functions:

» It builds and maintains the outer layer of cell membranes
» It determines cell membrane permeability (decides which molecules can pass into the cell and which can not)
» It is involved in the production of sex hormones (estrogens and androgens)
» It is essential for the production of hormones released by the adrenal glands (*like the stress hormone cortisol*)
» It aids in the production of bile that helps digest fat
» It converts sunshine to vitamin D
» It is necessary for the metabolism of fat-soluble vitamins (A, D, E, and K)
» It insulates *nerve fibers*
» It builds *brain cells*

Cholesterol is carried through the blood by molecules called "lipoproteins." That means it is a compound that contains both a fat (lipid) and a protein. There are three types of lipoproteins:

» **LDL (low-density lipoprotein)** is referred to as "bad cholesterol" because excess amounts form harmful buildup of plaque along the walls of arteries, causing narrowing and decreased blood flow to the heart. Think lard, bacon grease, French fry oil, etc.

» **HDL (high-density lipoprotein)** is referred to as "good cholesterol." This is the "good oil" you want for your Ferrari. This oil lubricates the arterial walls but does not form plaque. Think olive, flax, and coconut oil—as well as avocados and raw almonds.

» **Triglycerides** are dangerous fats that remain in your blood. They are formed from carbohydrates, excess calories, alcohol, and sugar that are eaten but not immediately needed for energy, so your body converts them to triglycerides and stores them in fat cells. Triglycerides are only released from fat cells when there is no other source of energy available, like in the case of fasting or famine. But most of us are not fasting and have never had to survive famine. This process is controlled by hormones and triggered by *stress*. If we continue to eat junk food, we continue to pack these triglycerides in fat cells around our middle.

*There is no such thing as good or bad cholesterol.* There is, however, good and bad oil. Let's simplify. If you eat a third-pound hamburger with two slices of "squirty" yellow cheese and a pile of French fries, that is bad oil, which creates LDL cholesterol. Any time you ingest the cholesterol of dead animals, processed cheese, and oils fried at high temps, you are clogging your arteries.

Good oils, such as cold-pressed olive oil in a glass bottle coat the coronary arteries and block calcification from occurring. Coconut, flax, avocado, hemp, and chia are other good choices. These oils do not stick to arterial walls. Calcification and narrowing of arteries is the main cause of heart disease.

Triglycerides are made from fats found in carbohydrates and junk food. Potato chips, cheese-flavored crunchy snacks, macaroni and cheese, candy bars, grains and sugars, doughnuts, and anything processed with hydrogenated vegetable oils are junk. These fats have no nutritional value, and if you are physically inactive, they end up being stored around your middle.

So what type of oil would you put in your Ferrari? Would you really feed your beloved family pet French fry grease and melted "squirty" cheese that just shouts, "Go ahead, clog my arteries"?

Ancient man stored excess calories as fat. This was and is a protective mechanism—hardwired into human DNA for the purpose of survival. Excess calories to ancient man were things like fruits, root vegetables, nuts, and seeds. These foods, when stored as triglycerides, could sustain ancient man for up to a month in times of famine, drought, or icy winters.

Modern man still stores excess calories as fat. The problem is that the carbohydrates we eat today are industrially processed and hydrogenated and would not even be considered edible by ancient standards. Things like doughnuts, cereal, or anything made with white flour and sugar need to be *eliminated, not stored,* within eighteen to twenty-four hours. When you eat too many of these high-calorie, nutrient-lacking foods, your body may reach its storage capacity. Your liver converts the stored sugars into triglycerides, or fats, so that the excess energy can be transported to the fat cells for longer-term storage. Your fat cells release this energy when needed. If you eat more calories than you burn, your body will continue to store the fat. *Adrenaline (a stress hormone) stimulates their release, while insulin inhibits them.* This is very important to keep in mind.

Carbohydrates provide almost instant energy. They break down into simple sugars that are absorbed in your gut and released into your bloodstream. If you are active and exercising, you burn these calories and utilize the sugar as energy. If you sit at a desk, or on a couch, and never exercise, within minutes your blood sugar level begins to rise. Your body in its infinite wisdom releases insulin. Insulin is the hormone messenger that allows sugar to enter fat cells for storage. As the sugar enters the fat cells, it is effectively removed from the bloodstream, your blood sugar level goes down, and your body is back in balance.

A diet high in carbohydrates (that break down into sugar)

causes your body to produce more and more insulin to bring your blood sugar level down. Eventually, your pancreas can't keep up with the demand, and you become "prediabetic." You may be told you have "insulin resistance" or "metabolic syndrome." Wouldn't it be logical then, that instead of taking synthetic insulin to keep up with the excess carbohydrate and sugar intake and lack of physical activity, to merely decrease your carbohydrates and start walking?

Our parents and grandparents knew the terms "hardening of the arteries" and "coronary heart disease." This was a feared disease that few talked about or heard about routinely on the nightly news. The term cholesterol is still feared, and few know how absolutely necessary good oils are for your entire body. Mostly what you hear from mainstream media and medicine are a class of drugs called "statins." **Statins Are Dangerous Drugs**

Remember, cholesterol has many crucial functions, as listed above. There is no such thing as good or bad cholesterol—only good or bad oils, a.k.a. raw material that you ingest and provide to your liver. What's a hardworking liver to do? It has no choice but to take what you give it and make cholesterol. This wonderfully made lubricating substance is in your bloodstream for protection; is what every cell membrane in your body is made from (all trillion of them); is found in hormones, vitamin D (cholesterol produced in your skin to hold moisture), and bile to digest fat; and helps coat nerve fibers and form memories in your brain.

Statin drugs are a class of drugs called HMG-CoA reductase *inhibitors*. These drugs *block* an enzyme in your liver that produces cholesterol. Any time you block or inhibit a natural body process, you are interfering with your natural cellular intelligence to maintain homeostasis. The enzyme that is blocked is CoQ10. *You must have CoQ10!* If you have a loved one or know of someone taking statins, please share this and suggest he or she asks a doctor about a good CoQ10 supplement. This enzyme is essential for the creation of ATP, which you need for cellular energy and mitochondrial health. Your heart obviously has the highest energy requirement and therefore requires the most CoQ10 for optimal function.

The goal of statin drugs is to reduce the overall production of cholesterol to under 4mmol/liter and 2mmol/liter for the LDL, and therefore treat and prevent atherosclerosis or narrowing of the arteries. But every cell in your body needs cholesterol, and since your liver produces it, forcing your liver to halt its production is not the answer. Even people with a family history of high cholesterol *still need good oil* to coat their arteries, or the acids they consume will burn a hole in them. The point is, putting good oil in your body is a smarter strategy than eliminating *all* oil. Statins block all cholesterol in an effort to reduce the bad.

Isn't that like punishing the whole class because one kid was misbehaving?

Blocking all production of cholesterol is dangerous and requires liver function tests every six months to make sure there is no liver damage.

*And there are even more dangerous side effects with statin drugs.* Statin drugs can cause high blood sugar, or hyperglycemia. When you force the liver to stop making cholesterol, you send the simple sugars back into the bloodstream, and as mentioned above, your blood sugar levels rise. That causes you to need more insulin to remove the sugar from the blood and store it. Increased workload on the pancreas means it eventually can't keep up with insulin production—so your doctor will think you have developed diabetes. Not true! You told your liver to disregard its innate intelligence by forcing it to stop production with a statin drug. Now you must artificially control homeostasis with statins *and* insulin. High insulin levels cause heart disease. Isn't this counterproductive? Did I miss the memo that we are trying to prevent heart disease? Your body will resist anything that isn't natural to attempt to bring you back into balance.

Statin drug-induced diabetes and having type 2 diabetes without being on statins are two different issues. If you are taking a statin drug, and your blood sugar is elevated, it is very possible you have a side effect of hyperglycemia as a result of the statin medication. Working with your doctor to get off the statin could normalize your blood sugar and prevent the need for insulin. Changing your lifestyle by adding in good, heart healthy oils, decreasing carbohydrates and junk food, and getting a little sunlight and exercise could get you off both!

The side effects of statin drugs should not be surprising when you consider the necessity of cholesterol and the fact that statins block production of it. *Muscle problems like rhabdomyolysis* (a serious degenerative muscle tissue condition) have to do with liver malfunction. This is the most common side effect. Chewing milk thistle seed helps this. Milk thistle is one of the best plants for your liver and can build muscle and even help with cirrhosis!

Statins can cause *polyneuropathy* (nerve damage in the hands and feet). Other side effects include anemia, acidosis, memory loss, sexual dysfunction, and pancreas and liver dysfunction.

Statins are considered a "pregnancy category X medication," which means they are a *known cause of serious birth defects*. Any woman planning a pregnancy should first work with her doctor to get off them!

Coronary artery disease is the leading cause of death in the United States. Heart and cardiovascular disease kill more people each year *than all cancers combined*.

Statin drugs are one of the top fifteen most prescribed drugs in the United States. They are a multibillion-dollar industry, even though most conventional medical doctors agree they have *no proven benefit* for most people and are particularly harmful to women. A Google search of "dangers of statin drugs" returns 2,300,000 hits in under half a minute. Websites like www.pubmed.com show many peer reviewed medical studies that have documented serious adverse effects. *Still, despite all that research, one in four Americans over the age of forty-five are prescribed statins.*

So let's recap:

» You are a middle-aged man or woman with hormonal changes and your digestion is slowing down.

» You have a sedentary lifestyle with moderate stress (remember—the stress hormone adrenaline shuts down digestion and releases triglycerides from fat cells for energy to prepare for fight or flight). This does not get rid of the fat storage cells around your middle, it just releases *sugar* stored in them back into the already sugar-overloaded bloodstream.

» All of this sugar and artery-clogging oil causes sluggish blood flow, and you are diagnosed with "high cholesterol."

» You are put on statin drugs.

» Your blood sugar levels begin to rise and you are told you are prediabetic, insulin resistant, or have metabolic syndrome.

» Now you take statins and insulin but still have fat around your middle.

» As your belly grows, you will probably be diagnosed with sleep apnea and put on a breathing machine because the fat around your middle blocks air flow when you lie down.

» Meanwhile, your partner is lying awake from the snoring and noise of the breathing machine …

In studies of populations with the highest longevity and lowest heart disease, participants who consumed cold-pressed olive oil in glass containers lived the longest and were free of heart disease. It may come as a surprise, but chocolate made from raw cacao was a big winner too. Please be sure you understand—this is not the same as commercially processed chocolate with white sugar and hydrogenated oil. This is my favorite raw chocolate: http://www. sacredchocolate.com/home.php

Juicing green leafy vegetables and celery builds blood, lowers blood pressure, and strengthens your cardiovascular system. The chlorophyll in green plants has, as its center atom, magnesium—which, along with the elements sodium and potassium, power your heart.

Coconut oil is very helpful in the prevention of Alzheimer's. There are many studies proving the benefits of coconut oil—most notably that of Dr. Mary Newport, who reversed Alzheimer's in her husband.

Hawthorn is one of my favorite herbs for heart health. Milk thistle is my favorite for liver health, as well as raw organic beets juiced or shredded in a salad. Vitamin D3 is very important to hormonal health. You must have D3—only D3 (not D2) is the natural form of the vitamin from cholecalciferol. Vitamin D2 is a synthetic, often ineffective form.

You need to reduce stress. Meditating works well. There is a popular homeopathic remedy appropriately named "Rescue Remedy" that helps calm and relax you. Rescue Remedy comes in several forms. If you suffer from chronic stress, this may help. Visit your local health-food store for more information.

You may want to ask your doctor about taking niacin or vitamin B3. You may need a prescription for this, though it's unlikely. Studies have found that vitamin B3 is lacking in people with high cholesterol and causes their blood cells to stick together. Vitamin B3 and fat cells are discussed in more depth in the chapter on PTSD (see chapter 13).

This might be a good time to mention that I am not paid to endorse anything that I mention as my favorite. I mention products only because I have personally tried them, trust their source, and would feel perfectly safe giving them to my own children or loved ones. My purpose is *not* to diagnose or prescribe. That would be the role of your medical doctor. Please keep in mind that you *must work with your doctor* when trying to make healthy changes.

Lifestyle changes, like adding good things slowly and with grace will help bring your body back into balance naturally and without side effects. Walking—even just a little at first—gets your blood flowing and brings oxygen to your lungs while getting rid of carbon dioxide. Singing does the same. Sunshine brings you energy and light. These simple changes, when added slowly and with grace, become good habits that bring heart health and longevity. Don't take my word for it—the best research is that which is done with your own eyes, your own ears, and an enquiring mind. Find your own personal truth.

Burton Goldberg said it best:

"Pull out the poison, feed the body, and God will heal."

## RESOURCES:

Links to my favorite products:

Blood purifier and builder:
http://www.herbsetc.com/ChlorOxygen-Mint-1-oz-AF_p_23.html

https://www.innerlightinc.com/www/ProductDetail.aspx?item=000241

Your liver will love Milk Thistle:
http://www.natureswaystore.com/product/milk-thistle-standardized-15171

http://www.mayoclinic.com/health/silymarin/NS_patient-milkthistle.

Your heart will love it:
http://www.luckyvitamin.com/p-4740-natures-way-hawthorn-standardized-extract-90-capsules.

Make sure your CoQ10 is orange-colored and is derived from "ubiquinone." I don't have a favorite source for this one.

Rescue Remedy:
http://www.vitacost.com/bach-flower-remedies-rescue-pastilles-black-currant.

## ADDITIONAL RESOURCES:

For more information about Cholesterol:
http://articles.mercola.com/sites/articles/archive/2010/08/10/
making-sense-of-your-cholesterol-numbers.aspx.

For more information about Statins:
http://articles.mercola.com/sites/articles/archive/2010/07/20/the-
truth-about-statin-drugs-revealed.aspx.

For more information about Dr. Mary Newport; here is her personal
blog and her TEDx talk about coconut oil and Alzheimer's:
http://coconutketones.blogspot.com.

http://www.youtube.com/watch?v=Dvh3JhsrQ0w.

Drug Watch is my favorite site for information about drugs:
http://www.drugwatch.com/search/?q=statin+drugs

chapter five

Connecting the Dots—
Liver, Cholesterol,
Hormones, and Low T

*Close your eyes. Fall in Love. Stay there.*
—Rumi

Most of my writing takes place either late night or late morning. Late at night is the only time I have peace and quiet. I am not an early morning person—even though I am forced to play one in everyday life in order to get my son out the door by seven o'clock. No matter how late I stay up, I always have lots of company on Facebook. Many of my women friends can't get to sleep or stay asleep. Meanwhile, many men sleep very well and snore really well too—thanks to breathing machines that make sure they breathe regularly all night long. Men blame our sleep problems on "hormones" but have no clue that hormones are responsible for their sleep issues as well.

A theme that will be repeated throughout this book is that in order to have vibrant health, you must understand how your body works at the cellular level! Most doctors are *clueless* about

*liver methylation. If they* had *a clue, they would abolish statin drugs!*
When your innate God-given youth (sex) hormones decrease, so
does quality of life—along with physical and mental decline, loss of
energy, loss of memory, and diagnoses of heart disease and arthritis.

Hormones run every function in our body. Hormone health
is *critical* to wellness, energy, and longevity. Hormones are the
chemical messengers that travel throughout the bloodstream
coordinating complex processes like immunity, fertility,
metabolism, and puberty. Many of these hormones are actually
*steroid* hormones—steroid meaning "body regulators made from
cholesterol." Indeed, it is the very feared substance we've been told
we must eliminate.

Remember cholesterol from the previous chapter? Cholesterol
is the basic building block of all steroid hormones, and it gives them
all a similar structure. When you look at a molecular diagram of
all the steroid hormones, they look almost exactly alike. This is
because they all originate from the natural breakdown of fats and
sugars. *Without enough cholesterol—say, because you are taking statins
and blocking production of it—you don't make enough steroid hormones.
That means you are deficient in the following hormones:*

» **Pregnenolone:** the steroid hormone precursor from which
all other hormones originate, very potent memory enhancer,
reduces stress, improves mood and energy, improves
immunity, reduces PMS and menopausal symptoms, and
repairs the myelin sheath (The protective coating around
nerve fibers). At seventy-five years of age, your body
produces 60 percent less than you did in your thirties. (Even
though natural Pregnenolone was successfully used as far
back as the 1930s for rheumatoid arthritis and autoimmune
disorders, it was discontinued when pharmaceutical giant
Merck introduced the synthetic version, *cortisone,* in 1949.
Soon after, the synthetic steroid hormones prednisone and
dexamethasone were introduced.)

» **Progesterone**: dominant female hormone that opposes estrogens, protects against cancer

» **Estrogens** (there are three—estradiol, estriol, and estrone): oppose progesterone and testosterone, regulate healthy metabolism, initiate weight gain, allow water and sodium into cells causing fluid retention and high blood pressure if unopposed, oppose thyroid (iodine supplementation has been proven to help reverse polycystic breast and ovary disease)

» **Testosterone:** dominant male hormone, also present in females, responsible for sex drive, opposes estrogen, anabolic steroid, protects against cancer; ancient cultures associated it with physical strength and willpower.

» **DHEA**: memory hormone (because of Pregnenolone), increases lean muscle mass, decreases fat, promotes strong bones, increases immunity

» **Adrenaline**: supports fight-or-flight response, increases focus, requires natural salt to function optimally, allows humans to stand upright

» **Cortisol**: helps us adapt to stress, stimulates appetite, improves digestion, improves mood, supports fight-or-flight response, stimulates circulatory system, muscles, lungs, and brain, fights leukemia and lymphoma

The plot thickens …

The transformation from cholesterol to hormones, and from one hormone to another, requires an *enzyme,* which in turn requires *vitamin and mineral cofactors.* Taking HMG-CoA reductase inhibitors (statins) has been associated with a reduction in CoQ10, an enzyme necessary for every cell in your body and most especially your heart. Most of these conversions take place in your liver—but also in your adrenal glands, ovaries, testicles, skin, brain, and retinas.

Dr. John R. Lee has written many books about hormones. Here is an excellent description from *What Your Doctor May*

Not *Tell You about Menopause*: "The production of hormones is a dynamic, fluctuating system, constantly responding to changing body conditions and needs. Hormones are the control messengers for a vast, interrelated, ever-changing network of organ-system commands. As such, they must be continually synthesized for moment-to-moment situational needs and likewise must be metabolized and removed from the system when no longer needed in order for their presence to fall as their need diminishes."

In other words, hormones tell your cells what to do.

The organ responsible for metabolizing and excreting hormones as they travel throughout the bloodstream is your miraculous liver. It goes without saying that adequate cholesterol and a properly functioning liver are critical to making, delivering, assimilating, and excreting all hormones. Hormone health is absolutely *crucial* to a vibrant, balanced life that allows human beings to fulfill their purpose. The steroid, or "sex" hormones are the key. When you're young and in love, all the good hormones oppose and balance the stress hormones. This is vibrant health.

When you enter puberty, you are at the peak of hormone health. The hormone *progesterone* is a precursor to both the male and female sex hormones: estrogen (which is actually not a single hormone but a group of three) and testosterone, as well as all the critically important adrenal cortical hormones (a.k.a. *stress* hormones). *Precursor means you must have progesterone to make all the other hormones.*

Progesterone is made from the sterol pregnenolone → made from *cholesterol* → made from the breakdown of fats and sugars → and converted by mitochondria (power stations inside the cells). If you have been reading these chapters from the beginning, lightbulbs should be coming on! All the dots connect. Your body is miraculous and functions perfectly and predictably—*naturally.*

If you are a young male, testosterone is at an all-time high. If you are a young woman, the form of estrogen known as *estradiol* is dominating your health. *Estradiol makes everything grow and proliferate.* This estrogen, along with the hormone progesterone is responsible for making babies. Mother Nature is perfect and aligns sex drive with sex hormones for the purpose of procreation. Progesterone maintains the lining of the uterus, allowing the fertilized egg to attach and grow. Any drop in progesterone levels or blockage of any of its receptor sites will result in loss of the embryo due to premature shedding of the uterine lining.

Progesterone is the precursor to testosterone and adrenal corticosteroids. In men, progesterone is synthesized by their testes to produce testosterone and in their adrenal glands to produce corticosteroids. Testosterone opposes estrogen. Testosterone protects nerves, brain and heart health, and increases bone density.

From age thirty onward, your testosterone levels begin to drop. Even mainstream media and conventional medicine now acknowledge the condition referred to as "low T." For most middle-aged men, this process occurs gradually, unlike menopause in females. But the effects are very similar. Men develop high blood pressure and are put on medications that have undesirable side effects, including impotence. Impotence does not equal vibrant health! Men are told they have high cholesterol and are put on statins. Testosterone levels drop; estrogen becomes unopposed and causes them to gain weight. The increased weight causes fat around their middle, which causes heart problems and difficulty breathing when lying down, which leads to sleep apnea. Both men and women must have sleep to digest stress hormones and perform immune functions.

As a woman ages, she will still make estradiol, but as the production of eggs in her ovaries decreases, so does the hormone progesterone. As menopause nears, she will not make progesterone because it is secreted by the uterine lining after ovulation. But she isn't ovulating. Just as in men, this leads to estrogen dominance because progesterone balances estrogen and testosterone. This is a big problem for women and is becoming a problem for more and more men as well. Remember that estradiol *makes everything grow and proliferate.* That's great if you want to make babies—but a whole different issue if you are older than fifty and menopausal! Hmm … wonder what would grow and proliferate at that age—fatty cysts and tumors perhaps—as in PCOS (polycystic ovary syndrome)?

Progesterone protects the body from the undesirable effects of unopposed estrogens. Estrogen allows water and sodium into cells, causing water retention and high blood pressure. Estrogen opposes thyroid function, promotes histamine release (causing allergy symptoms), decreases the amount of oxygen present in cells, promotes blood clotting (which increases the risk of stroke and embolism), thickens bile and promotes gallbladder disease, causes loss of zinc, copper retention, decreased sex drive, increased risk of fibrocystic breasts, uterine fibroids, endometrial cancers, loss of bone density, and prostate cancer.

Young girls, in the peak of sexual health, are choosing to take birth control pills at an earlier age, and delaying childbirth. *Birth control pills are synthetic, laboratory-created estrogens. Young men are taking synthetic steroid hormones.* Synthetic testosterone, estrogens, and laboratory created "progestins" have a different molecular structure than natural hormones made from fat. As these molecules travel the bloodstream, they fill up estrogen and progesterone receptor sites in the reproductive organs and glands, but *the body does not have the enzymes and cofactors to metabolize and excrete them.* Synthetic progesterone does *not* have the innate ability to make estrogen and testosterone like natural progesterone. *These synthetic hormones do not break down in your liver.* Therefore, it becomes a *toxin* that your body must remove from your blood and store in fat—mostly around your middle. Is it any wonder so many young girls are getting the same fat around their middle as middle-aged women?

Synthetic estrogens feed estrogen-sensitive tissues in your breasts, endometrium, uterus, and cervix. This *out-of-control tissue growth* begins as an estrogen waste product that can't be properly metabolized in your body because it is unnatural and toxic. The molecular structure isn't the same. Your body, in its miraculous wisdom, surrounds toxins with lymph to provide "crowd control" and stop them from traveling to distant sites and forming more *clusters of toxic tissue* (a.k.a. cysts and eventually tumors). Lightbulbs yet?

This same phenomenon occurs as women reach menopause. HRT (hormone replacement therapy) was first introduced in the 1960s using only synthetic estrogen. Thousands of women lost their lives after taking these unnatural estrogens from out-of-control tissue growth (a.k.a. uterine [endometrial] cancer). It took two decades of these trusting women dying needlessly before the mostly male medical profession realized unopposed estrogen was the cause. Unfortunately, the same medical profession spent the next decade in intense marketing campaigns and public relations spots convincing women that HRT was now safe and they would be protected from cancer with the addition of the synthetic hormone progestin— marketed most commonly in a pharmaceutical compound called Provera. This may have helped balance unopposed estrogens, *but synthetic hormones still could not be broken down in the liver like natural hormones.* So, again, your body removes them from the blood, surrounds them with lymph, and stores them in fat. The only way to remove toxins from fat storage is to stop putting them in your body and to lose the fat around your middle. Bioidentical hormones are much safer than synthetic hormones and in fact should be the only thing you take, but they only work as long as you take them. So you would have to take them for the rest of your life to continue to get the effects, which, considering the alternative, doesn't seem like such a big deal.

Since the 1940s, approximately *seventy-seven thousand chemicals* have been introduced to the human race. These synthetic, laboratory-created chemicals from petrochemical, industrial, pharmaceutical, and electrical industries were never intended for human ingestion. These chemicals are estrogen imposters called "xenoestrogens," which invade our cells and steal our estrogen receptors. There is no way for any human to avoid them. Industrial wastes pollute our air and water—food additives, pesticides, hormone- and steroid-injected meats in our food supply, and cell phones, computers, and electrical devices have stripped our world of healing negative ions and caused electromagnetic pollution. Electromagnetic pollution is becoming such an issue that many European countries ban cell phones for children ages five to eighteen. Most people are now aware of many of these toxins—fresh paint, dry cleaning chemicals, printing chemicals, ant killer, PVCs, dioxins, DDT, Benzene, parabens and phthalates in cosmetics, BPA in plastics to name a few—but are clueless as to how to limit them or prevent them from establishing a community around their waistline. Remember, in order to remove these toxins, you must stop putting them in your body, remove the fat in which the already ingested toxins are stored, and give your body the fuel it needs to perfectly and innately balance hormones.

In order to process and excrete hormones, your liver must be able to carry out the process of *methylation*. Methylation is the process of taking a single carbon atom and three hydrogen atoms, known as a methyl group, and finding a methyl donor to complete the chemical structure that allows hormones to perform their critical functions. Methy ($CH3$) groups facilitate reactions in your body. This includes making important critical substances like creatine, coenzyme Q10, melatonin and many others. Many critical body functions are dependent upon the ability of your liver to carry out the process of methylation. One function of this process is to remove bad estrogens, because by definition they are missing a methyl group. Methylation also turns on and off genes, fights infections, and repairs DNA. Methylation problems can be genetic—about 10 percent of humans have a deficiency of methyl groups and die of liver or heart disease in their fifties *specifically of that lack of methyl groups.*

This may sound complicated—but perhaps an example will help.

Western medical doctors test you for HDL and LDL cholesterol levels. The protein in the blood is *homocysteine*. Studies show that too much homocysteine floating around in the blood causes fatty deposits to stick to the arteries (atherosclerosis), which leads to blood clots and strokes. Homocysteine is missing a methyl group. In order to pull excess homocysteine out of the blood, it needs a methyl donor. The B vitamins—B6, B9, B12 (methylcobalamin) are methyl donors that grab these proteins, and with the help of the enzyme "methyl transferase" make the most active form of folate in your body, known as methylfolate. Without the B vitamins, zinc, and magnesium, this process can't be completed.

How important is folate? Methylfolate deficiency will cause toxic buildup in your bloodstream of the protein homocysteine. Methylfolate is also known as glutathione, which is the master antioxidant of the bloodstream. (You can get natural glutathione from good-fat rich avocados!)

The Mayo Clinic website lists all the conditions associated with folate deficiency: alcoholism, hyperhomocysteinemia (an abnormally high level of homocysteine in the blood), megaloblastic anemia, neural defects in pregnancy, Methotrexate toxicity, acute lymphocytic leukemia, Alzheimer's disease, arsenic poisoning, chronic fatigue, and depression.

Yet nowhere on the website do they explain *liver methylation*! Trust me—you have to do your research to connect the dots. You must have B vitamin methyl donors and essential minerals to pull out excess bad estrogens and homocysteine proteins from the blood.

There are many natural ways to add methylators to your diet. Here are a few of my favorites:

» **Raw Organic Beets**—juiced or eaten raw on salads, beets are trimethylglycine (an organic compound found in plants) and are liver methylators. If you are not juicing, you can buy beetroot (betaine) powder and eat it or add to smoothies.

» **Broccoli and Other Cruciferous Vegetables** are part of a group called indole-3-carbinols (I3Cs), which contain sulfur and methyl groups that act by educating your cells to produce proteins that bind to bad estrogens and remove them
» **Berries, Lemons, and Limes**
» **Glutathione** is a supplement and can also be found in foods like avocados
» **Vitamin D3**
» **Co-Q-10**
» **Natural Progesterone Cream**
» **Deer Antler Supplement**
» **Tongkat Ali Supplement**
» **Maca Root Powder (use sparingly)**
» **Coconut Oil** use coconut oil as much as you can in place of other oils for eating, baking, and frying.

**RESOURCES:**

Wolfe David. Longevity Now Conference, April 2011.

http://articles.mercola.com/sites/articles/archive/2000/08/27/adrenals.aspx.

Betaine Sources:
http://www.livestrong.com/article/291527-food-sources-of-betaine/

Explaining Homocysteine and Folate:
http://www.heart.org/HEARTORG/GettingHealthy/NutritionCenter/Homocysteine-Folic-Acid-and-Cardiovascular-Disease_UCM_305997_Article.jsp.

http://www.mayoclinic.com/health/folate/NS_patient-folate/DSECTION=evidence.

chapter six

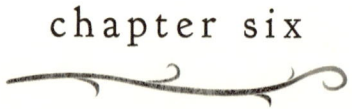

# My Transformative Journey Begins:

### Part 1: The Nurse

*To the question, "What does it take to be a healer?" Bernie Siegel (1986)*
*answers, "The willingness to deal with your own wounds."*
—Robbie Davis-Floyd, *From Doctor to Healer: The Transformative Journey*

When I graduated from nursing school in the early 1980s, I began working at our local hospital. Our floor soon transitioned to become the "cancer" ward or oncology department. In the space of two years, I admitted people who had pink cheeks and looked mostly healthy, and were full of hope that no matter what they had to endure with chemotherapy and radiation, they would emerge fully whole and resume their lives cancer free. There was a young boy with a brain tumor that caused frequent seizures; there was a retired nurse; and there was a young guy with a beautiful wife who had just recently given birth to their first baby girl. This particular guy waited all day for the doctor to bring him the results of his lung scan.

As I was getting ready to leave after working 3:00–11:00 p.m., his doctor finally swooped in and told me to get his chart and accompany him to the patient's room. We walked to the end of the hall and entered his room, and this doctor told the patient, "You have terminal cancer. I'll send the oncologist to see you tomorrow." And he walked out.

That was it. I left for home minutes later, still in shock, down the same hallway, passing by the patient's door. He was just sitting there on the side of the bed. I walked in and asked him if he was going to call his wife because she had been there earlier, anxiously waiting with him, but had to get home to take care of the baby.

He said, "No, I think I'll wait until tomorrow. She needs her sleep." I offered to sit with him but he said, "Thanks, I'll be okay." It was a scene often repeated.

How could he be okay? *I wasn't okay.* I went home and thought about him all night. I thought about the injustice of waiting all day for a doctor who had the compassion of a rock. I thought about his sweet wife and how happy they had been earlier that evening, talking about their new baby. His new baby. And I cried for them.

I cried for all of them. They were the kindest, sweetest, most decent people. They were never demanding. I held their hands through painful treatments, I held their heads through unbearable sickness, but mostly I watched these beautiful souls slowly become the gray, fragile shadows that cancer and chemotherapy leave behind. The healthy pink-colored faces, so full of hope initially, slowly faded to gaunt gray skin stretched over bone. One of my patients went quickly. As I walked in to give him his medication, he grabbed my arm and looked into my eyes and pleaded, "Help me." But he started hemorrhaging blood from his mouth and nose, and it was determined that his carotid artery had ruptured. He had been receiving radiation, and there was nothing I (or the code team) could do. When someone looks in your eyes and asks for help, but all you can do is hold the patient's hand and watch him die, you never forget it. It changes you forever. Trust me.

"Don't get attached. Keep your professional distance," my wise, well-meaning, older nurse mentors advised me, trying to protect me from letting it "get to me."

Sorry, girls, *no can do*. And any nurse who tells you he or she can is in the wrong profession.

It's one thing if you work on a maternity floor and everyone goes home with a baby, a cool little hat, and a token washtub. But how can you justify the fact that you are repeatedly putting chemicals used in warfare into people and telling them it will make them better? I could no longer be part of something I didn't *believe* to be true. I had to get out before I was required to become certified to give chemotherapy.

Nurses are trained to make careful observations, and there is no mistaking the look of cancer. And fear. And quiet resignation. And battle fatigue. Quality of life traded for quantity. These very faces became etched in my memory.

One woman I admitted refused treatment. She stood out from everyone else because she had the most unusual orange color. She explained to me that she was only there for tests and was headed to California to work with a doctor who believed in juicing to heal cancer naturally. She told me everyone thought she was crazy, but she had watched her mother die a slow and painful death from cancer and chemotherapy treatment, and she refused to do the same. If she was going down, she was going down kicking and screaming, not drugged out and defenseless! She refused to eat anything but raw food (mostly carrots), which explained her unique color. The oncologist and most nurses thought she was just "out there." But her valid research intrigued me. She was absolutely certain she could heal herself naturally with juicing. Her absolute *belief* and conviction resonated with me. So did her unwavering faith. She asked me to pray with her, and I asked her to keep in touch; I told her I would continue to pray for her, and I *believed* if anyone could beat it, she could. And she did. Cancer free.

Years later I was teaching a nursing skills lab at a local community college and working for an orthopedic surgeon. Eventually I was working twelve to sixteen hours daily at the office and had to give up teaching. I absolutely loved my job, my coworkers, and my boss! I had a cool sports car (300Z), my first house, money in the bank, and I was the personal assistant to a prominent orthopedic doctor who trusted me to write his orders and fill in for him in his absence. Life was good. But the hours were crazy. I never knew when I was going to get home or how long I would be there before I would get called back to the hospital to make rounds with my boss. Many times I would tell my husband I would meet him for dinner but not get home until midnight. He wasn't a fan. Or I would get a call at 11:00 p.m. from my boss, usually with a mouthful of popcorn, asking me to pick him up at 5:00 a.m. to make rounds before he went to surgery and I went to the office. You had to know him. We all loved him. But I was getting tired. And he got called to active duty in the Gulf War and closed his practice.

A friend gave me a bottle of an herbal preparation called "KM" that was formulated by Dr. Karl Jurak for his own specific health challenges in 1922 and distributed by Matol Botanical. I began researching each individual herb that was in the preparation. I have this insatiable hunger for knowledge and understanding. There was no Internet, no instant search engines—just bookstores. I bought a book and listed every property of each herb in the formula. It was an amazing botanical preparation. I traveled halfway across the country to meet Dr. Karl and hear his story. He had been working on his doctoral thesis in botanicals when he came up with this formula to purify his blood so he could climb the Australian Alps without becoming short of breath. Karl knew that climbing the Alps meant you tethered yourself to some friends, and if one of you became weak and slipped, you risked the lives of the others. Karl had done that and didn't want it to happen again and endanger his friends. He had been sharing his preparation for many years and helped thousands of people feel better. The more I learned, the more I knew the body would heal itself if given the proper nutrition. Dr. Karl was a brilliant scientist, a warm humanitarian, and a kind, caring man.

My neighbor at the time was your typical "sitcom" busybody. She was so crippled with arthritis that she would drive across the city street from her driveway to mine to keep me updated on the neighborhood gossip. I kept telling her about KM and how much it could help with all her ailments, and she kept telling me how much her knees hurt and the cost of all her medications.

One day when I was wearing my white uniform as always and going to work, she honked the horn and blocked my driveway and rolled down her window. "Are you a nurse?" she asked.

I laughed and said, "Yes, why?"

She said, "I just thought you were a quack or a hippie or something, always trying to sell me that herby stuff!" And she drove off.

She wasn't alone. Most people thought I was crazy. But I was so excited to find such a great product—based on *good science*—that I would tell everyone and go on and on and on …

To me, it was like finding gold in my backyard. I wanted to share it with my family and friends. So I'd say, "Hey, I found gold in my backyard! Come over and you can dig up as much as you want!"

And my family would say, "Uh, I have to work."

And my friends would say, "Uh, I don't have a shovel."

And I learned a valuable lesson. *You can't want something for someone more than that person wants it.*

In 2000, in a small town called Lone Pine, on the way home from a funeral, I listened to Tony Robbins talk about green drinks, Dr. Robert Young, and "live blood microscopy." This was the defining moment, the catalyst of transformation, right there on Interstate 79 in Lone Pine, Pennsylvania.

I don't believe in coincidences, because I believe everything happens for a reason. But I do believe in "synchronous events," which Dr. Siegel calls, "God's way of being anonymous." And a Divine hand was definitely guiding me toward natural healing. In *Physician in Transition* (1989), Peter Albright describes synchronous events like a "string of beads." At the time these events happen, they don't seem like steps in a process, but as you look back, you can string them together like a necklace.

In his book *The Recovery of the Sacred,* Dr. Carlos Warter states, "When these events occur, *we embark in search of our individual truth.* It is the undercurrent of the mystery of life that guides us and gives us the correct timing for our actions. Thus we need to learn patience, an important element in the larger context or 'big story' of our existence" (1994, xviii, emphasis added).

The next step was to begin studying for my doctor of naturopathy degree. I was ready. I was excited! I understood alkalinity and healing the body at the cellular level. I researched programs and found exactly what I wanted.

Just as I was about to begin, another event happened that would change my life forever. My husband was diagnosed with cancer.

# chapter seven

## My Transformative Journey

### Part 2: Cancer as a Blessing

The following is from one of my favorite textbooks, *Deep Healing,* by Dr. Emmett E. Miller. I can't speak highly enough of Dr. Miller.

### "God Games"

"The gods and goddesses of ancient Greece, I am told, once gathered on Mount Olympus to play one of their favorite games: 'Hide the Truth from Humankind.'

"'Let's hide it at the bottom of the ocean,' cried one.

"'No, he'll eventually build submarines and find it.'

"'How about up on the moon?' suggested another.

"'No, he is too ingenious for that. He'll eventually get there too.'

"Finally, the most mischievous of the gods, the one represented in humorous drawings as the little angel whose halo is always somewhat askance, spoke up. 'I've got a great idea. Let's hide it deep inside him. He'll never think to look there.'"

The book goes on to say, "I am told that there was great rejoicing on Mount Olympus that day, for they realized that, as civilization grew more and more complex, the resulting stresses would generate a state of mind so distracted that few would ever perceive the subtle nature of truth within."

But I didn't learn this until much later. First came the lesson and the "blessing" called cancer.

It all began in October 2001. My husband decided to have this "cyst" in his jaw removed. People had been noticing and commenting on his cheek, and the cyst appeared to him to be getting bigger and more noticeable. (He had planned to get it removed the year before, but my oldest son had broken his arm and spent a few months in physical therapy.) He made an appointment with a plastic surgeon near his office. I asked if he had checked credentials and recommendations.

He said, "It's just a simple cyst removal."

Evidently, the plastic surgeon felt the same way. He felt my husband's cheek and told him it was a simple cyst and he could remove it in the office the following Friday. No X-ray, no biopsy. At the time, I did question the fact that he didn't biopsy first, but I figured he was the surgeon (and must know better than the rest of us), and my husband had mentioned to him that he had had the cyst since he was thirteen years old—he was now forty-one. Surely it couldn't be cancer after all those years.

The nurse called and said my husband was ready to come home.

When I arrived he was still a little groggy, but he looked up at me and said, "I have cancer. The doctor wants to talk to you."

I said, "Are you sure you heard correctly?"

He nodded yes. I asked the nurse if she could please find the doctor because I had a two-year-old in my arms, and a nine-year-old to pick up at school twenty-eight miles away. She said she would try to find him for me and disappeared. My husband was still emerging from that abyss between anesthesia and consciousness, so I didn't ask him any questions and the nurse didn't say one thing or offer any details.

Forty-five minutes later she apparently was still looking for the doctor. For crying out loud, it wasn't a corn maze. You tell someone he has cancer and disappear?

I went to find her. She told me the doctor must have left and he would talk to us on Wednesday when we came back in for follow-up. She gave me one single pack of gauze and said, "They'll change his dressing on Wednesday, but in case you need to reinforce it, here is some gauze." I hadn't even met him but I already didn't like the bedside manner, or lack thereof, of the surgeon. I can understand and deal with complications, but this seemed like cowardly avoidance.

During the thirty-minute ride home, my husband attempted to recount what the surgeon had told him. He said that when the surgeon opened his cheek he found a little more than he expected and it was cancer, and that he'd had to remove it in pieces. They would send the specimen to a lab, and the doctor hoped to know more by the time we went back for a follow-up on Wednesday. Then he left.

My husband asked the anesthesiologist to show him what they had removed. He brought my husband a small container with a bunch of pieces of tissue floating in it. I didn't tell my husband that the worst thing you can do is remove cancer in "pieces" because you run the risk of one of them getting into the bloodstream and taking up residence somewhere else. I didn't have to. It wasn't good news at all.

And then there was the drainage tube incorrectly hooked up behind his ear. By the time we got home, his dressing was soaked and uncomfortable. There was no "reinforcing" it with the one piece of gauze they had generously afforded me. When I removed the dressing, I saw what appeared to be a straw coming out from behind his ear. Every time he swallowed, his saliva would come out of the top. If he smelled something cooking or even thought about food, it shot out of there like a squirt gun. It was genius really, with the mere mention of the word "steak" or "apple pie" and the correct aim, he could wipe out an entire table full of people with that thing.

I gave up on the gauze and just put towels on his shoulder. It was ridiculous. Needless to say it was a rough weekend with little sleep. We didn't say anything to anyone because we didn't know what we were dealing with. My husband stared at the fire in the fireplace and slept.

On Monday morning, the doctor's office called and asked to see us as soon as possible. We arrived and were told the doctor would be with us shortly. And then we waited. And we waited. Finally we were taken back to a small, dimly lit room, and after another wait, the surgeon and his senior partner came in. They looked like funeral directors about to tell someone a loved one had passed away.

Senior partner did most of the talking. It went something like this: My husband's cancer was a very rare aggressive form. In order to make sure they got it all, they needed to go back in as soon as possible. This time it would be performed in a hospital where they would remove the entire cheek to be able to fully see and explore the facial nerve and lymph glands. They would remove the lymph glands and check the nerve all the way back to the base of the brain to be sure no cells had "spilled" during the first surgery. They would then remove a skin flap from his back to replace the cheek, and sew his eye shut until they could be sure the facial nerve was working. He would be in the hospital for three weeks—if there were no complications. If the lymph nodes they removed had any cancer cells present, they would also do radiation. Hopefully, within three months, he could return to work. Oh, and by the way, the skin on your back doesn't match the skin on your face, so they could hook us up with some medical-grade makeup that my husband would have to wear for the rest of his life.

One word kept going through my mind: *no*. I thought, *This can't be happening.*

My husband was close to tears and in total shock. He asked Senior Partner about statistics. "You have a fifty-fifty chance of surviving two years." That did it. My husband totally shut down.

He told me later that all he could think about was not being able to watch his boys grow up. I saw the complete hopelessness in his eyes. Which lead me to one of things I tell all my clients.

*Statistics are facts about somebody else.*

No doctor has any business telling anyone how long he or she has to live. No doctor is God, or worse yet, a Mayan historian running out of stone tablets. None of us are promised tomorrow. Which brings me to my second mantra—

*Only* God *is* God.

My husband and I have been together since we were in high school. He has never been afraid of, or backed away from, anything. Except for a brief stint in middle school as a "hack man" for the basketball team, football was his game. His favorite line: "Ah, nothing like the sound of crunching a quarterback." He was the All-State defensive lineman. He is not a man I could ever see wearing makeup. He was paralyzed with fear and completely shut down with helplessness. In his mind, he was already dying.

Western medicine promotes this paranoia. Words like "victim" and "survivor" imply that cancer chases you down a dark alley with a gun and you are *powerless.* That couldn't be further from the truth. But there are distinct advantages to the victim mentality. You can look outside yourself with the illusion that the control of the situation is out of your hands. This is the *biggest roadblock to both healing and cure.* In order to heal at the cellular level, you have to look deep *inside yourself.*

But first I had a few pressing questions for Senior Partner.

» Was this standard procedure for this type of cancer? "Yes."
» So no matter where we would go to have it done, they would still remove the cheek, sew the eye shut, and remove the lymph nodes? "Yes."
» Would you mind if we got a second opinion? "No, not at all."
» Will you be doing the surgery? "Yes."

» Have you had any other cases where you performed this surgery? "Yes, two of them."
» Are they still alive? "Sadly, no."
» Sadly, no, you will not be performing this surgery on my husband.

To be honest, Senior Partner really seemed sincere. Or maybe he was just determined to cover for his partner. I don't mean to sound ungrateful. He was very kind. And he had beautiful skin. (I almost asked him about moisturizers.) But because of the actions of his younger partner, I really wasn't sure if they were being truthful, or if they really needed to go back in there because the first surgery had gone so wrong. I think that the young, cocky surgeon got in way over his head. Why else would you leave someone with a "squirt-gun" ear?

They wanted to operate that Friday. That was just a little too soon for me. I told them we needed time to process this information. They told us they had to send the cancer specimen to an army lab for further tests because it was so rare their lab couldn't classify it.

In the car, my husband said he just wanted to get it over with and was ready to stay local and have it done in four days. But I wasn't. I needed to do some research. But first I had my most dreaded task of all. I had to tell my nine-year-old son that his dad had cancer.

My firstborn son was an only child for seven years. And before Xbox, video games, ice hockey, and cell phones, there was going to fire stations with Dad, camping out with Dad, learning to fish with Dad, and a hundred GI Joe adventures with Dad. My son had a GI Joe figure for all of us—even a nurse for me! They staged battles and took pictures and made their own GI Joe videos.

When I arrived at his elementary school, I ran into my dear friend, who reminded me about the PTA meeting that night. I told her I couldn't be there. She asked what was wrong, and I broke down. I told her what we had just found out and she hugged me and cried with me. The beautiful women friends of mine in that PTA were my strength. I heard that there were lots of tears at that meeting. They organized people to bring us meals, added us to their church prayer lists, and offered to stay with my antisocial two-year-old who cried when anyone looked at him sideways. Friends we hadn't heard from since high school sent notes or prayed for us. This love and support meant the world to me.

The only thing my son remembers is the exact location of the car when I told him. He was worried but okay. It was hard to see his dad lying there on the couch staring at the fire, withdrawn from all of us.

Later that night, when everyone was asleep, I looked up "adenocarcinoma of the parotid gland" on the Internet. Indeed, the surgical procedure seemed to be the same. One doctor in England seemed to be considered an expert, so I e-mailed him and explained what we had been told and asked if he had any advice. He was very nice and e-mailed me back. But the verdict didn't change, nor did the procedure. I wondered if I was just in denial. What if I had to accept that this mutilating surgery was the only way?

By now I had been juicing for almost ten years. I wore out my cassette that came with my "Juiceman" juicer, by Jay Kordich. I was drinking a green drink periodically and I owned the book *Sick and Tired: Reclaim Your Inner Terrain*. I was receiving a newsletter from a distributor of Dr. Young-created products named Steve. I knew Dr. Young was a great microscopist and alkalizing was good for your blood, but it never occurred to me this could help with cancer. This was all pretty new to me, and I was just beginning to understand. I didn't know Steve and had never met him, but he seemed to know Dr. Young and sold his products, so I asked him if he knew what specific products Dr. Young might recommend for cancer. And then I fell asleep.

The next day, Steve e-mailed me back and sent me an article about a guy with stage-4 lung cancer who had beaten the odds by following Dr. Young's program. He didn't know what specific products he had used, but Steve asked me, "Why don't you call Dr. Young and talk to him? He does consultations." *Seriously?*

Two days later I was anxiously preparing for my phone consultation. Remember, this was almost eleven years ago. I was still in "nurse" mode. I gathered the few test results and lab reports that I had in case he had questions, and called Dr. Young.

He didn't need to know any of that. He asked me one question: "Is your husband ready to take responsibility for his health?"

*Yikes! I wasn't ready for that one.*

At first I was a little surprised at his matter-of-fact attitude. There was no pity in his voice. There was only strength of conviction. There was no hesitation, and he was absolutely certain my husband had to change his diet and alkalize his blood. My specific concern was losing those lymph nodes. Lymph tissue is a blessing. It surrounds foreign bodies to stop them from multiplying and migrating. I asked Dr. Young how long my husband needed to be on the greens before his lymph nodes would be clear. He said two weeks. I had my answer. I knew what to do. Dr. Young was so absolutely certain about his research that he gave me the confidence and the unwavering belief that in two weeks there would be no trace of cancer in those lymph nodes.

I tried to explain it to my husband, but he wasn't processing much. The only thing he remembers me telling him was, "Give me two weeks, and you'll be okay." And we immediately changed our diet and went green. I ordered "Supergreens" and several other products Dr. Young recommended.

The cloud had lifted for me. Dr. Young empowered me to be the rock, when everyone else was crumbling. And to be honest, I was on my own. People listened to me extol the virtues of Dr. Young and alkalinity, but no one seemed convinced. I always got the silence and blank stares. I talked to my old nurse buddies from the hospital, thinking they would be excited for me, and their response was: "You know that natural stuff doesn't work. The cancer always comes back somewhere else." That hurt me more than ever. As if cancer never came back after they administered chemotherapy? We both knew the answer to that.

The only person who believed in me was my nine-year-old son. One of his fourth-grade teachers was interested in telescopes and stargazing. So at night after his brother went to sleep, we told his dad we were going outside to "stargaze." We would sit on his swing set and talk about his concerns or fears about cancer. Once I explained the theory of alkalizing the blood, he instantly knew his dad would be okay. We built a whole GI Joe mission around taking care of our wounded soldier. He drew pictures of "green" army men in tanks and planes attacking cancer. He gave his dad a little green army man to keep in his pocket to remind him that we were all with him and he was strong. I asked him to try to keep his dad laughing. All his fourth-grade classmates wrote notes and jokes to "Mr. C."

A lot of people told my husband to get a second opinion. In fact, his boss called and talked to me about going to Johns Hopkins in Baltimore. We live fewer than two hours from there. I totally agreed. So did my husband. We also got some good news from the army lab. The cancer was not the deadly, aggressive kind but instead was a slow-growing type called "acinic cell carcinoma." Senior Partner said the surgery would still be the same.

We tried to get an appointment at Johns Hopkins on our own, but they said it would be weeks. We asked Senior Partner if he could call for a referral to Johns Hopkins, and we were able to get in the following week. I can't say enough about Johns Hopkins. It is a totally different atmosphere and an amazing, healing place. The surgeon there asked my husband to get an MRI locally and bring it with him to the appointment.

By the time we went to Johns Hopkins we had completely changed our diet. Specifically:

» We ate no meat—but I did use Boca Burgers on occasion.
» I made fresh juice every day with apple, lemon, carrots, beets, and a pound of greens—Dr. Young would not have

approved of all the sugar (apples, carrots, beets), but it was the only sugar my husband was doing at the time. I made juice based on my Jay Kordich tapes and Dr. Norman Walker book.

» My husband super hydrated with two products called Supergreens and Prime pH. He drank about two gallons of water a day with a scoop of Supergreens and Prime pH in each gallon.

» We ate a lot of raw broccoli with olive oil and sea salt, fresh homemade hummus and celery, cauliflower "mashed potatoes," and Ezekiel-brand sprouted grain bread.

» He took a few additional supplements initially (for detox) that were recommended by Dr. Young.

I saw a huge change in my husband. He was interacting again. He went back to work with his "special diet": a gallon of water and a pack of washcloths for his trigger ear. His skin cleared up and years of fungal nails grew in normally for the first time. His blood pressure was great, and he lost about twenty pounds. Of course all the doubters thought the weight loss was because he was getting sicker. At a time when he was supposed to be so ill, he looked and felt the best he ever had. And even though we had been together for many years at this point, we were closer than ever. For the first time, my husband really paid attention and didn't continually think about work.

The surgeon at Johns Hopkins was fabulous. He examined my husband, looked at his chart, and had talked to Senior Partner about the previous surgery. There was a lot of conflicting information regarding the previous surgery. At one time, they had said they got all the cancer, and then they said they got half the tumor and there was another half under the facial nerve. The MRI showed a spot near the surgery site that the surgeon couldn't really determine, without going back in, whether it was inflammation of the lymph nodes or cancer cells left behind. So my husband was given the following options:

» Do nothing and wait. (This was my personal favorite.) Since the cancer was acinic cell and slow growing, we could wait and hope they'd gotten it all, and we were just seeing inflammation.

» He could do one round of radiation. But you could only radiate this area once and then that would no longer be an option.

» He could go back in and "clean up" the area to be sure there was absolutely nothing there. Cleanup involved an incision along a natural crease in his neck that would barely be noticeable afterward; he would fold back the cheek and explore the facial nerve down to the base of the brain and lymph nodes closest to the previous surgical area. He would have the first and closest lymph node tested for the presence of cancer cells. If there was no cancer in the first lymph node, he would leave them all. *I loved this man!*

This was approximately a two-hour procedure, and my husband would have to stay overnight. He had an opening in his surgery schedule the following week. I asked the doctor if he had ever heard of Dr. Robert Young. He had not. I told him we were alkalizing and doing green drinks and he wasn't going to find any cancer in those lymph nodes or elsewhere. I got that same old roll-the-eyes look and a smile. Yes, sir, I am one proud *quack*!

My husband was absolutely convinced he needed the second surgery. When he saw all those pieces of his tumor after the first one, he felt for sure there were many more still left inside. So he opted for the cleanup surgery. There was only one more question to ask. Would he still have this annoying tube in his ear after the next surgery? The doc laughed out loud. *Sadly, no.*

So there we were. November 27, 2001, approximately twenty-one days after the first surgery, and my husband was laughing and only slightly nervous. The students were observing and helping him get ready. They asked us if they could have the tumor to study back in the classroom.

I said, "There won't be anything in there."

The surgeon laughed and told them, "His wife has him on some green diet."

We signed a paper allowing them to take the specimen to study. My husband was more than happy to donate! I headed to the waiting room.

Two hours seemed like an eternity. And still I waited. I tried to read magazines, but nothing was registering. I paced. I began my typical "what if" scenario in my mind. What was taking so long if there wasn't anything in there? What if I had been wrong and the cancer had spread? This was an awful lot of pressure for a novice!

Finally the surgeon emerged and sat down next to me. He said something like: I just spent the last half hour going over this with your husband, but I doubt he will remember any of it. I explored the lymph nodes and sent a piece of the first one to the lab to be tested. There was no cancer. Just to be sure, I sent a second one. There was no cancer. There was no inflammation. I checked the facial nerve all the way back to the base of the brain. There was absolutely no cancer. In fact, I found absolutely no cancer cells anywhere.

I wanted to "go televangelist" and jump up on the furniture and shout "Hallelujah!"

We later learned that my husband's surgeon was called before the cancer tumor board to ask why he'd operated on a man who clearly had no cancer.

In November 2011, my husband was released from Johns Hopkins after ten years of follow up. He remains cancer free, medication free, and recently helped some skinny state trooper push two people stuck in a jeep a quarter mile out of the middle of the road to safety. He didn't know the parking brake was on the entire time!

## RESOURCES:

My favorite books on cancer:
http://cancerbooksource.com/defeat-cancer-book/

Radical Remission is my all time favorite!
http://www.radicalremission.com/index.php/about/the-book

My favorite cancer M.D.:
http://www.connealymd.com/

https://www.youtube.com/watch?v=73dJEsM57-E#t=13

Free video series:
http://thecuretocancersummit.com/video-series-enter/

chapter eight

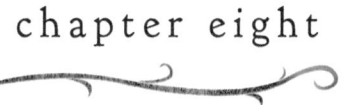

# After Cancer—Normal Becomes Extraordinary, Part 3

*"Aren't You Dying to Start Living?"*
—From the song, "Feel" by my favorite musical group Chicago

I often wonder what might have happened if my husband would have opted to have the surgery performed locally. The very word cancer evokes such fear that people are willing to accept without question the antiquated, limited options of mutilating surgery, chemotherapy, and radiation. Get rid of this stuff as soon as possible—no matter the long-term consequences—because no one thinks about long term. And why does the medical profession feed this fear and refuse to educate themselves about current, well-researched, and well-documented scientific *proof* that cancer is being reversed, defeated, and cured *now*?

To this day, my husband will not talk about his experience with cancer. Integrating back into "normal" is very difficult even after you are declared cancer free. The fear of it coming back is always lurking. A simple runny nose makes you wonder. Everything changes. At the same time there are many lessons. We learn who really matters, and we remember "don't sweat the small stuff, it's all small stuff," and most of all, gratitude for breath, another sunrise, one more band concert, and love. Fear is incapacitating. Love is healing.

David Wolfe talks about how doctors and patients are programmed by old thinking. He mentions a book by Thomas Kuhn (1962) titled *The Structure of Scientific Revolutions*. Wolfe says that often times scientific theories can be so entrenched in society and protected by the Ivory Tower of medical practitioners, people no longer even question their validity. And perhaps society may have actually gotten so far on an incorrect assumption that it was never questioned. Take Louis Pasteur and his germ theory. Western medicine continues to operate under this false belief that germs cause disease. On his deathbed, Pasteur himself admitted, "I have been wrong. The microbe is nothing. The terrain is everything."

Eventually, evidence is so profound that is contrary to popular belief, or even violates the walled-up Ivory Tower theory; and this evidence becomes available in such an abundant and undeniable way that the walls of the Ivory Tower crumble and the old theory falls apart. But Western medicine is so *slow* to embrace leading-edge science that it takes at least fifteen or twenty years to penetrate and change the academics (professors) of medicine that decide what will be the "standards of practice." And so, the standards of practice continue to be medieval and archaic. Doctors of naturopathy and integrative medicine, on the other hand, *know* cancer means your body is out of balance. Leigh Erin Connealy, MD, states: Your "inner terrain is in disequilibrium."

When you understand healing at the cellular level, cellular metabolism is the primary focus, rather than disease syndromes with scary names and individual treatment protocols. The cause of disease is cellular malfunction, which in turn is caused by two things:

» too much acid (toxicity)
» too few nutrients (deficiency)

Chemotherapy and radiation get rid of tumors, but they *do not get rid of cancer.* If you only treat tumors with chemo and radiation, you remove the tumor—but where does it go? It doesn't just evaporate. The cells go back into your bloodstream to be eliminated. If your immune system is strong, eventually it will eliminate the debris. But your immune system will not be strong if it has to keep fighting against toxins. All tumors begin as a single, sugar-hoarding rebel cell. Most experts agree it takes between two and twelve years from single cell to tumor. Chemo, surgery, and radiation break down tumors, but you still have circulating tumor and stem cells in your bloodstream. The biggest fear when my husband had his surgery and the tumor was removed in pieces was that one of those cancer pieces would spill into his bloodstream and head down toward the base of his brain.

Even if your scans are clear, you must get rid of these circulating cells in the blood to know the cancer is gone. How do I know this? Because these circulating cells are what your doctor measures as "cancer markers." Ever wonder why on follow-up your scans are clear, but the next time you go back your markers are up? Now you know why. Your body has not eliminated the circulating tumor and stem cells. You can do this naturally by detoxification. Learn more here: http://www.cancer.gov/cancertopics/factsheet/Detection/tumor-markers.

At the cellular level, the battle for survival is an epic one and played out in the river of life called your bloodstream. White blood cells, known as *lymphocytes,* defend your body from foreign invaders, cancer cells, and toxins. *Macrophages* are grownup white blood cells that attack and gobble up foreign invaders and cancer cells. Macrophage means "big eater." They essentially salivate or secrete substances called *cytokines* that scope out the battlefield. Cytokines decide how the immune system will respond—keep eating up all the garbage, or surrender. When macrophages are exhausted, they die on the battlefield. Your entire immune system will begin to decline—your natural killer (NK) cells and T-cell levels go down, your bone marrow dries up, and you won't produce B cells—the circulating cancer cells and chemo toxins will seize the opportunity to take over. Your pH changes from the packed acids and toxins and you lose your appetite because your blood is full of toxins. So wouldn't it be logical to stop adding toxins and instead recruit more soldiers? If you're pouring in toxins faster than you're building the soldiers to fight them, you're losing the battle.

Dr. Connealy, quoted above, says it best: "Blood delivers the groceries. Lymph takes out the garbage."

We all know what happens when garbage collectors go on strike.

Dr. Otto Warburg won a Nobel Prize in 1931 for his discovery that cancer cells only thrive in low oxygen. When your body cells and tissues are acidic (below pH of 6.5–7.0), they lose their ability to exchange oxygen, and cancer cells are able to thrive by the process of fermentation. Normal cells thrive in oxygen-rich environments. Cancer cells hate oxygen. There are alternative therapies based on that fact alone. Doctors have known about the importance of oxygen and alkalinity since 1931! They have studied Dr. Warburg's work and Nobel Prize work yet never tell a cancer patient about the importance of alkalinity.

This is why I immediately understood the scientific credibility of Dr. Robert Young. Dr. Young is a world-renowned microbiologist who practices and teaches a revolutionary technique to view live blood samples to identify nutritional deficiencies and acidic toxicity. It's like high school biology on steroids! From a single drop of capillary blood taken from your finger and immediately magnified on a computer screen, you can see exactly what is in your blood at this very moment. The characters are all there: red blood cells, white blood cells, parasites, cancer cells, etc. I have had it done twice. It is fascinating and scary. It forces you to accept the truth. You are what you eat. Live blood doesn't lie. Nor does Dr. Young. He is a brilliant scientist with impeccable integrity, who conscientiously researches and shares his knowledge. Never just take my word for it. Remember that the best research is that which is seen with your own eyes, heard with your own ears, and filtered with an open mind.

Here is an example of live blood, courtesy of David Wolfe's Longevity Conference. Watch the macrophage eat! http://www.youtube.com/watch?v=wpHRQg-v98A

When my husband was diagnosed with cancer, we were never told anything about pH balance. Dietary modifications were never discussed and in fact were dismissed as having no correlation to disease. I had no idea cancer cells feed on *sugar*. All carbohydrates break down into sugar. Soda is loaded with sugar. Some fruits are high in sugar—even carrots and beets are high in sugar.

The doctors ordered a PET scan. It was considered "experimental" at the time. Positron emission tomography is now a common test where a positron-emitting radionuclide (radioactive tracer) is paired with glucose and injected into your body through an IV solution. Then you wait an hour. Meanwhile, sugar-hoarding cancer cells gobble up the sugar. These sugar cells are radioactive and can be seen with a scanner. The tumors are illuminated. They are surrounded by sugar. This is how they see if your cancer has spread to other areas. The point being, doctors knew way back then that cancer craves sugar. This amazed me. How could they know this and still insist there was no correlation between diet and cancer? I mean, even Hippocrates, way back in 300 BC, said, "Let *food* be thy medicine."

In order for a cancer cell to take in abundant amounts of sugar, it has to form extra blood vessels to receive it all. These extra intake vessels or receptor sites have the appearance of crab legs and claws. A regular cell has four receptor sites. A cancer cell has ninety-six. *This is how it is able to overwhelm your immune system.* You would think that today, twelve years later, doctors would advise patients about sugar—but in my experience, this was not the case. Not only that, they refuse to acknowledge that diet plays any significant role.

Last summer I asked a radiologist about building bone marrow with wheat grass and the herb milk thistle. He dismissed me with a wave of his hands—as if I were a two-year-old—and told me that had "nothing to do with it" and recommended a popular pill with severe side effects.

*Stressful thoughts* of fear, anger, resentment, etc. set off a cascade of hormonal events designed to save your life. Remember, our stress response is designed to deal with eminent danger and produce fight-or-flight decisions. It is the role of the hormone adrenaline to remove/utilize glucose (sugar) from the body's cells for instant energy to either fight or run and then return to the pre-stress state. Prolonged stress causes a depletion of adrenaline. Depleted adrenaline causes a buildup of glucose in the cells and increased circulating cortisol (acid) to balance the adrenaline. This sets up the ideal environment for cancer cells to *thrive.*

All healing begins in your mind, with your thoughts. The subconscious beliefs we carry have the most impact. Your thoughts transmit to neuropeptides; neuropeptides bind to immune cells; all immune cells have a neuropeptide receptor; therefore, your thoughts become your immune system.

People who do not look at cancer as a death sentence; those who realize it is NOT something that comes from the outside and takes over their life; those who instead seek the answer within— beat cancer. The fact that you have a diagnosis simply means that you have become *aware* of something that has been imbalanced in your body for many years. Listen to your internal wisdom—it will never lead you astray.

Dr. Ryke Geerd Hamer did amazing work, with extreme scientific accuracy, proving 100 percent of the time by using brain scans that *all* cancers correspond to an unresolved emotional conflict. You must also do the emotional work to heal your soul.

Start by loving yourself. Unconditionally …

Following are my favorite resources:

You will find lots of therapies to help cancer patients work through these issues to heal. I love these books and videos! There are many treatment options and they are beautifully explained:

Miller, Emmette. *Deep Healing*, pgs. 207–245.
http://drmiller.com/meetdrmiller/story/

Strasheim, Connie. *Defeat Cancer*. This book will give you strategies from *fifteen* doctors who are successfully treating and defeating cancer.
http://cancerbooksource.com/defeat-cancer-book/

*Cancer is Curable NOW*.
http://www.cancerbooksource.com/cancer-is-curable-now-dvd-documentary

Dr. Young's new book:
https://www.phmiracleliving.com/p-632-the-ph-miracle-for-cancer.aspx.

Excellent information about the emotional causes of cancer:
http://www.alternative-cancer-care.com/dr-ryke-geerd-hamer.html.

Just to summarize and add a few details:

**Exercise**—According to the DVD *Cancer is curable NOW*, exercise is mandatory and reduces cancer by 50 percent and is like "chemotherapy without side effects." (Quote by Dr. Leigh Erin Connealy, MD. Link above.) Make it fun!

**Oxygen**—sing and chant out loud! Stop fermenting! "Take each breath that's given to you, to love back the ones who love you!"

**Sunlight**—you must supplement with *Vitamin D3! It has to be D "3"*. Everything else is synthetic. And go sit in the sun for a little while— but please don't put gobs of sunscreen on or you will block the healing rays.

**Reduce Your Stress**—what makes you happy and peaceful? Meditate, pet your dog, walk on the beach, listen to music, and try yoga or Qigong or doing more of what you love.

And never ever give up! There are many people who have lived "happily ever after" despite incredible odds. Here is one story: *Dying to be Me* by Anita Moorjani. http://anitamoorjani.com/

Here are many other stories of remission:
http://www.harpercollins.com/9780062268754/radical-remission

Extra articles for further reading:
http://www.nobelprize.org/educational/medicine/immunity/immune-detail.html.

http://www.news-medical.net/health/What-are-Cytokines.aspx.

http://www.cancer.gov/cancertopics/factsheet/Detection/tumor-markers.

# chapter nine

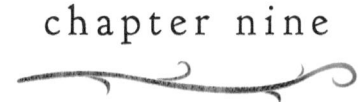

# Stand Guard at the Door to Your Mind

*If you correct your mind, the rest of your life will fall into place.*
—Lao Tzu

Certain themes will be woven through all chapters and explored. Obviously, the first theme is that your body is miraculous and has the innate ability to heal itself. In order to heal your body, you must become more alkaline. All disease begins when your pH consistently falls below 7.0 in the acid range. You could say that acidity is the "smoking gun." *Stress* is the trigger.

You can eat the best food and drink the purest water, but if you are starving emotionally, it won't save your life. You can have fame, money, the best doctors, expensive cars, and homes all over the world, but if you are angry, frustrated, or fearful, all the drugs, alcohol, and antidepressants will not save you. No one can slay your dragons but you.

You have to make a conscious choice to stand guard at the door to your mind, and control your stress. Hans Selye is credited with defining stress. There are three stages a person goes through when responding to any type of stress (bad or good—like riding a roller coaster):

1) Alarm: this is the initial phase where your body recognizes a threat to you and begins the fight-or-flight response. The stress hormones *adrenaline* and *cortisol* are produced.
2) Resistance: in this stage the body attempts to adapt to a threat, which is persisting. This requires physiological resources and adrenal hormones, which can become depleted if the threat persists
3) Exhaustion: if the perceived threat to the body lasts too long, your immune system breaks down, and long-term damage and sickness occur.

Stress for ancient man was much different than the stressors faced by modern man. For ancient man, adaptation to stressors was a necessity for survival. Stress was a short-term physical emergency. He had *physical* stressors like predators, famine, and temperature extremes. The goal of physical survival is instant energy to the brain and muscles. One of the first hormones secreted is adrenaline, which supports fight-or-flight responses and is also responsible for keeping vertebrate bodies upright. Adrenaline release triggers two important responses:

» Oxygen supply and energy-giving glucose (sugar) to the brain and muscles is increased.
» *Bodily processes not vital to immediate survival are suppressed.*

But modern man isn't running. Or starving. Or freezing.

Modern man is sitting in rush-hour traffic or at a computer, listening to the evening news, worried about paying his mortgage, paying for college, caring for spouses or elderly parents with dementia, cancer, or Alzheimer's—all of which are *psychological* in nature. Naturopathic doctors looking at the cause of disease find a huge body of evidence to suggest that stress-related disease develops because modern man activates a physiological system designed to respond to immediate physical emergencies, not long-term chronic psychological or social issues.

You have just set in motion a cascade of hormones and a release of sugar that is now circulating in your bloodstream with nowhere to go. Remember, when you are in fight-or-flight mode, bodily processes not vital to survival are suppressed.

**Stress shuts down digestion.** No time for a candlelight dinner or stop at the drive-through when you are running from a predator! This is why you should never eat when you are stressed or upset—it causes acid indigestion.

In *Conscious Eating* by Gabriel Cousens, he says, "A stable emotional environment helps to gain clarity on the effects of what one eats. If one is centered and calm before eating, eats in a peaceful environment, and pays full attention to the food, the digestive process will be different than if one is emotionally upset, depressed, or angry and tries to eat during the stress of an important business luncheon, for example, or while reading the newspaper or watching the TV news."

**Stress shuts down reproduction.** Need I explain why you don't have time for this? In males and females, sex hormone production is slowed down or halted. In the case of physical stress such as running from a predator, a baby belly would slow you down, and a female would not be able to sustain a pregnancy. Remember, we are talking about survival of the species. So your body, in its miraculous intelligence, shuts down reproduction. In the case of famine, or temperature extremes, the baby would be in danger as well.

**Stress shuts down your immune system.** When you activate the stress response, all of your energy is focused on saving your life. Your body can't mount an adequate immune response when your energy is directed elsewhere. This is what happens during the stage of exhaustion—your hormones are depleted and you have excess sugar, both of which your body can't eliminate fast enough, because your stress is chronic and long term and you keep releasing them into your bloodstream.

**Stress shuts down your kidneys.** During times of stress,

your heart rate, blood pressure, and breathing increase to rapidly deliver oxygen and glucose. You must have adequate fluid volume in your blood vessels in order to accomplish this. Your brain sends a message to your kidneys to hold on to the water. The hormone vasopressin has the ability to block urine formation and regulate water balance. Your kidneys are remarkable bidirectional organs that can hold or release water to your bladder. Once released to your bladder, it can't go back.

Chronic stress affects every cell and organ in your body. It is easy to see how chronic stress directly contributes to hormonal imbalance and depletion, and the accumulation of excess sugar. If you are continually mobilizing energy from glucose instead of storing energy from live sources like the sun and raw food, you become sick and tired—your immune system becomes weak, and cell renewal and repair will cease. Without knowledge of how to strengthen and restore your energy, your body begins to age and you develop degenerative diseases like diabetes, obesity, and arthritis. You essentially dry up and decompose—it's the natural order of life.

The ancients spent lifetimes studying the art of longevity and the cultivation of energy. Chapter 22, "The Three Treasures," explains this ancient, sacred Daoist philosophy. But once again I'm getting ahead of myself.

# chapter ten

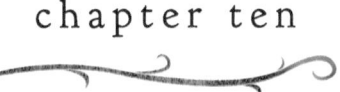

# Beyond Epidemic: Stress, Diabetes, and Obesity

*The first wealth is health.*
—Ralph Waldo Emerson

T he year my husband had cancer, my oldest son landed the role of "Dean Yule," the male lead in the fourth-grade Christmas play. Thanks to my high school pal and incredible music teacher, the songs were beautifully choreographed and performed. We were very grateful that my husband survived two surgeries in less than a month, was cancer free, and able to attend and enjoy it. My fellow PTA moms made delicious food that would impress even Martha Stewart. In fact, we always had an abundance of homemade goodies at the Halloween, Christmas, and Valentine's parties. One of my favorite things we did to raise money was to have a "Santa's Workshop," where the kids could buy gifts for their parents that cost no more than five dollars. The kids loved it, and we had lots of fun figuring out how to squeeze the most gifts out of the least amount of money. I still have my angel that my son picked out for me.

By the time my youngest son was in fourth grade, seven years later, there was no party at all. Some elementary schools had parties, but they were called Fall Harvest and holiday parties. No more "Christmas" or "Santa." Due to the *obesity epidemic*, treats were not allowed to be homemade and had to be prepackaged and "healthy."

Because let's face it, those fancy treats made by PTA moms three times a school year were responsible for the obesity epidemic. Shame on those cupcake-toting moms!

At the same time, my son was not allowed to carry around his personal bottle of water unless I brought in a doctor's note saying it was a medical necessity. And because our schools were so overcrowded, gym class was reduced to forty-five minutes once a week.

Lunch/recess was thirty minutes. There was no talking to your friends during lunch—teachers were monitoring to make sure you were eating quickly so they could "herd" everyone outside to run two laps in the hot sun with a stomach full of undigested food.

The last two minutes were yours to do whatever you liked.

And thus the obesity epidemic was solved. *Not.*

Obesity, stress, and diabetes *are* epidemic in our country. Diabetes is now pandemic. There are many contributing factors responsible for the huge increase. One thing is certain. The biggest contributing factor is lifestyle. Historically, diabetes mellitus was considered a disease linked to the lifestyle of the Western world. But as fast-food chains began to urbanize indigenous cultures and people around the world adapted to lifestyles of industrialized nations, the statistics changed. Perhaps even more troubling is the sharp rise in diabetes and obesity in children.

According to an article published online by Dr. Mark Hyman, here are some disturbing statistics: (link to article below)

» 1 out of every 4 kids have diabetes or prediabetes.
» From 2000 to 2008, the number of teenagers aged 12 to 19 with prediabetes or diabetes rose from 9 to 23 percent.

» 1 out of every 7 "normal" weight kids has prediabetes or type 2 diabetes.

» 1 out of 3 children born after the year 2000 will become diabetic.

Dr. Mark Hyman is a popular guest on the *Dr. Oz* show and has written many books, including *The Blood Sugar Solution*. Dr. Hyman talks about "skinny fat people" who are "normal weight but metabolically obese with all the same risks of disease and death as the obese." If you've been reading along so far, you should have some idea of why this is the case.

Skinny does not equal healthy. Remember that your body protects you by removing all acidic toxins from your bloodstream and storing them in fat deposits. If you are a skinny person, these fat cells develop all throughout your gut and surround your abdominal organs. If you are eating a diet that is mostly artificial, processed food, getting little or no fresh air or sunlight, and sitting around all day, your belly will be full of fat.

Remember too that *stress causes hormonal disruption.* Your hypothalamus is the major control center of your endocrine system. Your endocrine system is responsible for setting a safe weight for you, letting you know when you are hungry, and deciding how much fat to store or burn. The hypothalamus, like every other organ of your body, is driven by protection and survival. Survival is driven by *stress hormones.* Fat helped us survive famine and ice ages. It wasn't designed, however, to protect us from the powerful and global food industry.

In 1971, President Richard Nixon was facing a tough reelection campaign. The war in Vietnam was extremely unpopular, and food prices were rising. In order to appeal to the powerful lobby of farmers, Nixon hired an agriculture expert from Indiana, Earl Butz. If you think one person can't make a huge difference, think again. You might say this man was single-handedly responsible for the transformation of our food supply, not only in the United States but globally.

Butz quickly transformed American farmers from local multi-crop producers, to multimillion-dollar businessmen with global markets. He did this by pushing farmers into the massive industrial-scale farming of one crop. *Corn.*

Corn made everything "better." Cows were fatter, burgers were juicer, corn oil was cheaper for frying and baking. So Nixon succeeded in getting large quantities of cheaper food to the American supermarket, and farmers were getting rich in the process. By the mid-1970s, however, all this corn created a surplus. So Butz was once again called upon to travel to Japan to study a scientific innovation that would forever transform the food we eat.

Butz learned that the Japanese discovered a process for the mass development of *high fructose corn syrup.* High fructose corn syrup wasn't new, but the process to mass-produce it was not engineered until this moment in the 1970s. This one discovery literally changed our food supply overnight. High fructose corn syrup from surplus corn was cheap. It made everything better! It made everything sweeter! It extended shelf life from days to years!

And thus, the obesity epidemic was born. *For Real.*

In the fifties, when my grandfather operated his Nehi Bottling Plant in Steubenville, Ohio, I often heard my brothers talk about the process of bottling the soft drinks. They had huge bags of sugar and had to be very careful to keep the area clean and swept so that bugs and roaches didn't get into the sugar supply or worse yet, my favorite drink, Nehi grape soda, and ruin the product.

In 1984 in the United States, the Coca-Cola Company made the decision to switch from sugar to high fructose corn syrup at the risk of altering the taste because high fructose corn syrup was two-thirds the price of sugar. Other soft drink manufacturers quickly followed their lead.

During this whole process of dumping high fructose corn syrup into everything we ate and drank from the 1970s to the mid-80s, another health issue was looming. Heart disease was increasingly becoming a problem, and fierce debate over the cause was being researched in American academia. This time, instead of the farmers lobby, the sugar industry came out with blazing guns to make sure their precious high fructose corn syrup was *not* fingered as the culprit. *Fat was blamed instead.* The food industry again sensed huge profits to be made from the creation of a whole new line of products to save us from heart disease: "low fat" and "fat free."

Well bless their hearts.

Unfortunately for them it tasted like garbage. So they remedied that problem by adding more sugar.

And still we got fatter. We ate tasteless, fat-free food. We joined gyms. We put our kids in every after-school sport program imaginable. We limited our calories and joined weight-loss programs. As our middles became bigger, we started hearing about "cholesterol" and "triglycerides," insulin resistance, metabolic syndrome, and fatty livers.

Meanwhile, "lab rats" everywhere were puzzled by their expanding waistlines. Those who watched their diet and ate "rat food" maintained a normal rat weight. Those who were fed *processed high sugar content* food gained weight almost overnight. The more sugar they ate, the more they craved it. Their desire for sugar was insatiable. They too tried the whole calorie-limiting thing and the extra laps around the old wheel, but alas, as long as they ate the sugary stuff, the weight gain continued. They were *addicted*.

Most of the food we eat is nothing more than processed flour and sugar, the wrong kind of fat, and artificial flavors and colors. And the effects of these poor food choices are literally cutting years off the lives of our children and predisposing them to chronic diseases at earlier ages. This is not natural.

According to the above-referenced article by Dr. Hyman, here is what the average American eats per year:

» twenty-nine pounds of french fries
» twenty-three pounds of pizza
» twenty-four pounds of ice cream

» fifty-three gallons of soda
» twenty-four pounds of artificial sweeteners
» Almost three pounds of salt
» Ninety thousand, seven hundred mg of caffeine
» Forty-two pounds of corn syrup

We need to teach all kids about real food and good nutrition. But even more importantly, we need to start, before the baby is born, with the health of the mother. If the only energy you have ever heard of comes in a can you buy at a convenience store, then so too will your children. If your children are overweight and you limit their calories by buying "low-fat" or the "100 calorie" packs of cookies or crackers, they are still putting junk in their bodies with no nutritional value. And if you read the labels on those so-called "low-fat" foods, you'll find they are actually filled with artificial ingredients that you can't even pronounce and are worse for your body than the regular ones.

What if we could teach and empower children with healthy choices they grow themselves? What if we could show preschool children how to grow a beautiful sunflower sprout that opens its arms (leaves) to the sky and absorbs the sun's energy; makes beautiful green "blood" and stores it; and gives that healing energy to us as a gift when we eat it? What if we could teach high school children that the periodic table is not some outdated material to memorize but that each of us is made of C, H, $O_2$, and Fe, and by taking in these live, vital nutrients we can end ADD, ADHD, depression, diabetes, and obesity? Then health will become more than the absence of disease, and children will have vital energy to run, swing, play—and enjoy life.

There are wonderful programs that teach children just that. One of my favorites is Jones Valley Urban Farm in Birmingham, Alabama, where they have "seed-to-table" programs. Schoolchildren are taken on field trips to learn all about how seeds are planted and cared for and are then made into beautiful meals from fresh fruits and vegetables that they just picked, and they get to eat right there at the farm. Edwin Marty had a dream of turning a drug-ridden inner city block into a place of beauty and education. The food grown on the farm is shared with local food banks as well as sold on the farm to help pay the operating costs. You can find the link at the end of this chapter.

Another one of these programs was put into place after Hurricane Katrina and a documentary was made about it. It's called *Nourishing the Kids of Katrina*. Look for it on YouTube.

There is a growing movement to use whatever space you have to grow your own food and create your own garden. If you live in a high rise, there is container gardening. In South Central Los Angeles, Ron Finley is transforming front lawns and roadside grass into gardens—proving that every one of us can make the conscious choice to not only secure our own healthy food supply but to teach others how to do the same. And you don't have to have a lot of money or lots of land. Ron is amazing! For more information, visit the link posted at the end of this chapter.

In order to have vibrant health, you must have live, raw food. Not 100 percent—but at the very least 51 percent. We have to reverse this trend of feeding our children junk food—or for the first time in history we will end up living longer than our children. One hundred calories of mini chocolate-chip cookies is not the same as one hundred calories of broccoli. Freshly made juices and smoothies have so much more nutritional value than those filled with high fructose corn syrup. Our children are worth the conscious choice and extra effort to choose health.

## RESOURCES:

Thanks to Jacques Peretti for his in depth and well-researched article, "Why our food is making us fat."
http://www.theguardian.com/business/2012/jun/11/why-our-food-is-making-us-fat

*King Corn* is an excellent documentary on how corn changed the food industry. Look for it on YouTube.

Dr. Mark Hyman article:
http://drhyman.com/blog/2012/05/22/skinny-fat-people-why-being-skinny-doesnt-protect-us-against-diabetes-and-death.

For information on the Jones Valley Farm:
http://blog.al.com/spotnews/2011/04/jones_valley_urban_farm_founde.html

Here is a program developed to feed kids after Hurricane Katrina:
http://www.nourishingthekids.com

For more information about Ron Finley:
http://www.ted.com/talks/ron_finley_a_guerilla_gardener_in_south_central_la.html

## chapter eleven

# New Year's Resolutions and Diets—Just Say No Thanks

T he slate is clean, the page is white, and a new year stretches out before us. What choices will we make and what lessons must we learn? How exciting to expect this year to be the best yet to come! The canvas is blank, and the brush is in your hand.

I hope you will choose to live *consciously*. I hope you will choose to nourish your mind, body, and soul. Let's start with your mind— remember, that is truly where all healing begins.

When you tell yourself you can't have something anymore because you are on a diet, your body immediately senses that you are *lacking* something or *longing* for something you can't have. *Lack* equates to famine, and famine elicits the good old stress response, hardwired into your DNA to ensure survival. Anytime your subconscious mind perceives stress, lack, or famine, it goes into fat storage mode. Your body loves you. It is always trying to preserve you and keep you safe. Fat storage equals safety and safety equals survival.

No diet plan, no matter how well conceived or how many celebrities endorse it, is designed to work for you personally. It is not about counting things or assigning points (yay, no math!) or attaching labels like "vegan" or "raw" food only. Each one of us is biochemically unique and has to listen to our own intuition. Each of us, at various stages of our life, has different nutritional needs, different hormonal issues, and varying levels of stress, all of which affect our digestion and assimilation.

Human beings, ironically, with the most highly developed intellect, are the only species who seek the advice of others to tell them what they should intuitively know about themselves. Animals have instinct. You never see a squirrel seeking advice about how many nuts he should store as winter approaches. He doesn't loathe his thighs. He doesn't assign point values to walnuts versus stolen peanuts from a bird feeder. Squirrels eat naturally. No artificial ingredients. No peanut butter cheesecake. That's why you never see elderly squirrels shuffling along the power lines with orthopedic shoes and a walker.

Conscious eating is a lifestyle choice, not a diet. Diets are restrictive and depriving. When you eat consciously, you begin by slowly and gracefully adding good food. You change your mindset from the notion of, "I *can't* eat that anymore, I am dieting," to "I *can* eat anything I want to eat, and I *choose* to eat food that makes me feel great, healthy, and alive!" It is just a simple shift in attitude, but to your subconscious mind it is the difference between *lack* and *deprivation,* and *conscious choice.* Change the way you feel about things and a massive paradigm shift will occur.

You can't continue to send messages of lack and deprivation and expect your body to feel energized and alive. Stop self-loathing and begin loving yourself enough to take care of your body. Remember, your body is the earthly home of your eternal soul. Feed it well. Tell yourself this is a great thing you are doing and imagine how energized and alive you are going to feel! Get excited! Feel the difference? Or would you rather feel sorry for yourself because you are going to stop putting things on your fork that no longer serve you?

Conscious eating does not mean merely switching from

"regular" calorie junk food to "low-fat" or "gluten-free" junk food. If you read the labels, many times low fat is worse because they have to add more sugar or some other artificial ingredient to make it taste remotely palatable. And please—don't even get me started on artificial sugar! Replacing regular soda with diet soda will not help your diabetes! Even mainstream medicine knows that now, even though newscasters and the medical doctors they interview admit they drink several diet sodas a day in place of meals. Artificial sugar is toxic to your nerves (a.k.a. an "excitotoxin"). It doesn't matter what they name it—it is poison. That is my truth. Please do your own research! Replace soda with something like Kombucha, a lightly effervescent fermented drink of sweetened black tea. One simple change can make all the difference. A good habit is as easy to develop as a bad one. You will feel amazing!

Start adding organic fruits and vegetables. Yes, *organic*. It's not "elite"—pesticides cause cancer. Period. Support local farmers and buy grass-fed meat. Add God-made food that has proven super-nutritional value.

Grow some wheatgrass. Try liquid chlorophyll. Add lemon to your water. Research maca and pine pollen. Use coconut oil instead of butter. Make your own toothpaste and facial scrub with coconut oil and baking soda. Experiment. Make kale chips. Try Chia seeds and water in place of eggs. Try chia waffles for breakfast. Make your own whipped cream with full-fat coconut milk. Add a green smoothie.

*Try juicing.*

Begin where you are. Don't wait for a specific day or time of year. The pressure to start on January 1 causes stress. Start gently and gracefully. Add one good thing. And another. Be grateful for everything. Always focus on *adding* the good stuff. Never say or think thoughts of *lack*. Consciously choosing God-made, natural food will eventually make you feel so much better than eating junk food that you will no longer want it. Teach your children. Talk to your grandparents.

*Love yourself.*

chapter twelve

# Emotional versus Conscious Eating

Today is the day I refocus my energy on conscious eating. The holidays are over, my children are back in school, and the decorations are safely tucked away. My Pilates machine is back in place and quite stark in comparison to the twinkling lights of the Christmas tree. It is such a different feeling than just three short weeks ago when I was eagerly anticipating the magic of Christmas. But I am ready. Photos remind me of the beautiful memories I was blessed to share and the gift I was given of one more Christmas with the people I love.

If you are one of those people who have no emotional connection to food, this may not resonate with you. But for most of us, emotional eating begins in our childhood years, frames the way we eat, and subconsciously determines our relationship with food for the rest of our lives.

The only real reason to eat is to provide the raw nutrients to build blood cells and fuel your body. If you grew up in a large Italian family like I did, the homemade preparation and sharing of food meant so much more than that and was associated with family, love, traditions, comfort, and safety. A "chubby-cheeked" child was a healthy child, and anyone who didn't have a good appetite and "mangia!" was promptly taken to the doctor. It didn't help that the food was out-of-this-world delicious! My grandmother catered Italian weddings.

I was the baby of the family and the only girl. I felt very loved by my three older brothers and my mom and dad. I was always singing Beatles songs and climbing trees, and I was happy and smiling. I had amazing imaginary friends! People loved to pinch my chubby, rosy little cheeks and give me cookies and candy.

I went everywhere with my dad. His family owned a cigar store across from the train station in Steubenville, Ohio. I loved the smell of that store. It was a mix of cigars, candy, chewing gum, newspapers, and perfume. My aunt was always impeccably dressed in heels, cashmere sweaters, pearl jewelry, and lovely smelling perfume. I loved to watch her push the buttons on the gigantic cash register. She would let me pick any candy I wanted and sit in the big picture window out front and watch people at the train station come and go. When I grew up, I wanted to be just like my aunt and play with that cash register and wear makeup and pretty clothes.

Another favorite place was DiCarlo's Bakery. Since our families were friends, sometimes, even after the downtown store would close for the evening, I was allowed to go in with my dad or uncle through the back door. In the back of the store were huge troughs of bread dough rising, and ovens filled with baking bread. The smell of freshly baked DiCarlo's bread was beyond amazing. Ask anyone who grew up there and you will hear the same thing. I loved eating warm bread fresh from the oven.

Ann DiCarlo would take me to the front of the store and give me beautiful Italian cookies. I always got to pick one to eat, and then she would give me a box to take home. They were so delicious and sprinkled with all the colors of the rainbow and tasted of vanilla, almond, and anise. The sights and smells are forever etched in my memory.

My dad passed away when I was in kindergarten. I still remember the exact moment I was told he had died. I was listening to a silly song called *Never Smile at a Crocodile* (from the Disney cartoon *Peter Pan*) and getting ready for school. And just like that, he was gone. My first experience of pure, unconditional love, my big teddy bear of a dad, my favorite lap to curl up in, was gone forever.

Every time I went past DiCarlo's Bakery and smelled that bread, I was instantly transformed to a four-year-old holding my dad's hand in the dark alleyway and opening that back door to the warmth and smell of that bread. My mother died when I was eight, and I moved away. But every time I went home to Steubenville I would visit Ann DiCarlo and she would give me a cookie to eat and a box of cookies to take with me. I so loved those cookies. For me, they represented so much more than flour and sugar and colorful sprinkles. They represented a time in my life when I felt safe, secure, and loved.

Emotional eating is trying to fill a void that can never be filled with food. We all have our "voids"—loss, abuse, loneliness, boredom, pain—as well as our associations of food with celebrations, joy, coming home, and feeling loved. When I lost my parents, I lost the unconditional love that only your mom and dad can provide. Being so young, I had no choice but to go live with my aunt and had absolutely no control over the situation. I had to leave behind everyone and everything that ever meant anything to me. Food, in the form of cookies, was my effort to hold on to and stay connected to the happy childhood I was forced to leave behind. Cookies were my "happy," my comfort, my connection.

It wasn't until the birth of my first child that I finally felt unconditional love once again. And it wasn't until my husband had cancer that I realized how good it felt to eat for nutrition; how amazing and energized and light and happy I felt when I became alkaline—and how unconsciously I had been eating all my life.

Whenever I felt stressed or hurt or angry, I shoveled in the cookies. Or chips. It could have been cardboard. The more I replayed the exchange of harsh words or feelings of "what's wrong with me? I'm not good enough," the faster I shoveled in the food. Perhaps certain emotions trigger you to do the same.

It has taken me a long time, but I am finally at the point where I don't eat when I feel stressed. More importantly, I try not to allow myself to get stressed, even though, inevitably, there are days and times that I do. It was only by helping other people see this that I saw this in myself. Eating junk is easy. Doing the emotional work and looking inward is not. But you *must* do the emotional work to heal.

This is why I believe in the concept of conscious eating—as opposed to any other one-size-fits-all plan. In my experience, small yet powerful changes, made slowly and with grace, become good habits, which become a healthy lifestyle. Don't make it a big deal or make some big declaration on some huge holiday. This sets up unrealistic expectations, which lead to feelings of failure if you don't live up to those resolutions. Conscious eating allows you to find what works for you.

A simple change of habit like switching from coffee to Dandy Blend or Teeccino herbal coffee substitutes will break the habit without giving up the taste. A simple switch from white pasta noodles to zucchini noodles will satisfy your craving for pasta. I promise I never suggest anything I haven't personally tried or that doesn't taste amazing. I never liked pasta or store-bought sauce because it never tasted like my grandma's. Zucchini noodles with sun-dried tomatoes, garlic pepper seasoning, and olive oil come as close as you can get.

And even though I am very much against artificial sweeteners—I have yet to find a natural one that I would recommend—the herb stevia is considered natural, though I have tried to find a flavor I like. Honestly, it tastes sickeningly sweet and leaves a bitter aftertaste. Also be careful of brands like Truvia, which over-process stevia and create a product that is anything but healthy. In the words of "Food Babe" (who runs a highly popular blog about all things natural and organic), "The forty-step patented process used to make Truvia should make you want to steer clear of this stevia product alone, but there are two other concerning ingredients added (not only to Truvia but other stevia products as well). First, erythritol is a naturally occurring sugar that is sometimes found in fruit, but food manufacturers don't actually use the natural stuff. Instead they start with *genetically engineered* corn and then go through a *complex fermentation process* to come up with chemically pure erythritol." Visit her website for the complete article. (See link at end of chapter.)

I do like coconut palm sugar or honey. The point being— experiment and find what works for you. It is a learning process. Make it exciting! Imagine all the amazing recipes and new ideas to be explored. Knowledge is empowering.

Loving yourself is critical. This has been the most difficult lesson for me. You will never fill an emotional void with anything external and physical. Remember, it's not about dieting, giving anything up, or deprivation. It is a lifestyle. It is about choosing real food that nourishes you. It is about letting go of old traumas and chronic stressors that led you to poor food choices in the search for comfort. It's about consciously choosing food that makes you feel energized and alive, and letting go of foods that no longer serve you. There will never be a perfect time. Start with today, with where you are, and decide to make this the best year ever.

## RESOURCES:

These three resources are excellent for further exploration of conscious eating vs. emotional.
http://www.barnesandnoble.com/w/conscious-eating-gabriel-cousens/1100378932?ean=9781556432859

http://www.thegabrielmethod.com/free-chapter

http://www.hungryforchange.tv

Food Babe and a Report on Stevia-Based Products:
http://www.100daysofrealfood.com/2013/04/25/stevia-food-babe-investigates

## chapter thirteen

# Healing Leaky Gut—Bacteria: They Do a Body *Good*

In the movie *Stuart Little 2*, Snowbell the Cat delivers one of my favorite lines after coughing up a "major hairball": "And still we lick ourselves. Unbelievable!"

I often think of that line as people continue to put food into their bodies that they know will cause them "issues" later. Why would you choose to eat half a tub of ice cream if you know lactose gives you enough gas to power a lightbulb? Do you suffer from frequent heartburn yet still continue to eat foods you know you will trigger it? You're not alone …

The following stats are from the book *Integrative Gastroenterology* by Gerard E. Mullin.

» More than fifty million American adults experience frequent heartburn.
» More than three million children in the United States have food allergies.

» IBS (irritable bowel syndrome), which afflicts more than twenty-five million Americans, is the most commonly diagnosed GI disorder with *half of all patients dissatisfied with conventional treatment.* The most common cause of abdominal pain in children (especially recurrent) is IBS.

» Proton pump inhibitors (PPIs) like Prilosec OTC and Nexium are the third best-selling class of medication in the United States.

The problem with taking proton pump inhibitors for indigestion, or any other medication that acts by "inhibiting" or "blocking" a natural function, is that they *substitute* a pill for a *function* that your body performs naturally. By doing this, you override your innate, natural intelligence that knows perfectly and exactly how to heal itself. If you suffer from "acid indigestion" it is because you don't have *enough* digestive juice to neutralize the processed chemical artificial "food" and drinks you are taking in.

Natural foods that are not "cooked to death" come with their own digestive enzymes. If you eat them slowly, in a state of gratitude, you will not get acid indigestion. The body is always seeking balance. The opposite of the sympathetic nervous system, which governs the fight-or-flight response to stress, is the parasympathetic nervous system, which operates independently to "rest and digest." Stress shuts down digestion; rest enables it. The best way to digest stress hormones is to sleep. By miraculous design, your digestive system winds and curves to allow you to slowly absorb and metabolize the nutrients you choose to put on the end of your fork, and to get rid of waste within eighteen to twenty-four hours.

In contrast, true carnivores in nature skip the gratitude and go right for the meat—because they *have* to eat quickly before their meal runs away or a bunch of buzzards show up with forks. The digestive system of a wildcat, for example, is one straight tube— four times shorter than a human one, and his saliva is almost pure acid—the better to digest you with, my deer.

Early man ate naturally and seasonally. For the most part, humans lived peacefully in communities, shared meals, and grew their own food in dirt that was rich in minerals and nutrients. Gardens and eventually farm crops were varied and rotated, so as not to strip the soil of vital nutrients. Food was shared. Animals grazed peacefully on real grass and provided raw milk and antibiotic- and steroid-free meat.

Babies were breastfed and held close by their mother—fed when hungry—not at predetermined times or by convenience from a bottle. The human body needs the minerals and nutrients absorbed by plants, energized by the sun, and stored as chlorophyll and all the colors of the rainbow to make red blood cells and build strong bone marrow. Breastfed children receive those minerals and nutrients from their mother. In the first few days outside the womb, it is also crucial for a baby to acquire healthy balanced gut flora from breast milk in order to develop a healthy immune system. If a child does not acquire this gut flora, then he or she will not be able to digest and absorb foods properly. Without healthy gut flora, a human body will forever have a compromised immune system.

Life and death to a large degree are dependent upon the establishment of healthy balanced gut flora in the first few days of life outside the prenatal gate. This is the true definition of *natural immunity*. Natural immunity is passed down from mother to child, and as the child matures, so does the immune system, as well as the genetic predisposition to resist infection.

Fast forward. Modern man and woman have the same biological body as our ancestors, but the environment, culture, food supply, and lifestyle have changed dramatically.

Modern man eats quickly—stressed out, rushing through meals. He buys food with a shelf life, totally devoid of live enzymes—manmade with artificial, chemical, toxic ingredients that totally destroy good gut flora. Our soils have been stripped of minerals and contaminated with pesticides. Modern man takes multiple medications that destroy gut flora. For years young women take contraceptives that destroy gut flora before becoming pregnant. Bottle-fed babies, who bottle feed *their* babies, did not get normal healthy gut flora from the start, and in the first few years of life, damage their already-damaged gut flora with numerous vaccinations that forcefully inject toxins directly into their bloodstream before their compromised immune systems could even mount a proper defense—that is, if they had healthy gut flora. Without healthy gut flora there is little or no possible defense. A child with a compromised immune system built from baby formula—which doesn't deliver the same healthy gut flora as breast milk—reacts to vaccinations in unpredictable ways. The research is overwhelming. In many cases, vaccines further damage the immune system, causing chronic bacterial and viral infections, and requiring multiple doses of antibiotics for ear and sinus infections, and treatments for asthma, allergies, and eczema.

Western medicine likes to compartmentalize disease. If you have asthma, they give you steroids and an inhaler to treat the lungs. If you have ear infections, they give you antibiotics and eventually recommend tubes be put in your ears. If you have arthritis, they inject your joints with steroids and eventually replace them. What if all those body parts could be healed simply and inexpensively by healing your gut? Wouldn't it be worth a try?

Perhaps one of the reasons Western medicine has been slow to understand the miraculous loop of tubing we call the small intestine is because they couldn't easily get inside it to visualize it. You can't get to it by lighted scope from the mouth or the colon. Anatomically it lies behind and between other vital organs, so exploratory surgery was risky. Unexplained bleeding was always "assumed" to come from the small intestine, after all other parts of the digestive system were viewed and thus able to be ruled out. With the development of the "pill camera," from a company in India called Given Imaging, doctors were finally able to see inside the entire digestive system. This brought about new research and new understanding.

Years before, however, researchers proved that the gut operated independently of the brain and spinal cord. In his book *The Second Brain,* author Dr. Michael D. Gershon talks about how the study of neurogastroenterology started with two investigators named Bayliss and Starling in nineteenth-century England. Bayliss and Starling isolated a loop of intestine and found that the peristaltic reflexes that move food in one direction to the colon worked perfectly even without the brain or spinal cord.

Dr. Gershon explains: "For the reflex to take place in a system that contains no other organ but the intestine, all of the necessary elements have to be intrinsic components of the wall of the gut. This does not exist in any other organ. Cut the connections between the bladder, the heart, or the skeletal muscles and the central nervous system, and all reflex activity ceases."

This means your gut operates separately from the rest of your body and has everything it needs to do its job contained within itself. But what could you possibly need that you can only access from a small section of your approximately thirty feet of intestines?

Healthy gut flora. Happy microbes.

## Natural Immunity—It Does a Body Good

The key to eliminating many issues—autism, allergies, arthritis, chronic migraines, acne, depression, ADD, ADHD, PTSD, violent behavior, autoimmune diseases, obesity, fibromyalgia, restless leg syndrome—lies in the early acquisition of good gut flora— a.k.a. good microbes in the miraculous self contained world of your "second brain." There are more microbes in your gut than there are cells in your entire body. The gut is a highly organized microsphere, where good flora must outnumber and control the approximately five hundred species of pathogenic, low-frequency, opportunistic bad bacteria.

Dr. N. Campbell-McBride wrote *Gut and Psychology Syndrome,* in which she created the GAPS (gut and psychology syndrome) nutritional program in 2004 after working with hundreds of children and adults. Her discovery clearly proves a direct connection between the gut and the brain. Dr. Campbell-McBride found in her many years of research that almost all children with psychiatric problems and learning disabilities also have severe digestive issues. The book is an excellent resource, particularly for parents of children with behavioral or learning disorders.

The various functions healthy microbes perform are critical to vital energy and holistic healing. It goes without saying that the first function is digestion and absorption of nutrients from food. The best food, the strongest pill, the latest diet, or fat-burning craze will not work if it sits in your intestine and ferments. If you can't absorb and metabolize the things you choose to put on the end of your fork or in a drinking straw, you end up with multiple nutritional deficiencies and you don't feel energized and alive.

These are just a few of the deficiencies that are critical to fill if you want vibrant health:

» minerals like magnesium, zinc, selenium, iron (if you look pale and pasty and are possibly anemic), potassium, etc.
» vitamins B1, B2, B3, B6, B12; A, C, D3
» folic acid
» omega-3, -6, -9
» glutathione

How many of these vital nutrients have you heard of or seen in a health-food store? Any or all of these nutritional deficiencies are critical for the normal, healthy development of the immune system, brain, and body.

Healthy gut flora also act as housekeepers for the entire digestive system. When they colonize, they protect the entire surface of the gut from toxins and invaders. They provide a natural barrier by producing antibacterial, antiviral, and antifungal substances that nourish and strengthen the lining of the gut—*preventing leaky gut.*

Remember, with bacteria, it is always a matter of numbers. If you have little or no good gut flora, opportunistic pathogens have the opportunity to grow and colonize. If, for example, you have an iron-loving strain of bad bacteria growing in your digestive tract, it will consume whatever iron you ingest from your diet, leaving you iron deficient, and eventually anemic. Taking an iron supplement will only *feed the bacteria*, because without healthy gut flora, you can't absorb the iron, thus allowing the bad bacteria to grow stronger and increase their numbers. Make sense?

The research linking gut health to almost every chronic issue—neurological, psychiatric, autoimmune, and inflammatory—is undeniable. The fact is, most of your immune system, and 95 percent of the feel-good hormone serotonin, depend on the healthy functioning of your gut. Taking antidepressants that adversely affect your brain will not release serotonin in your gut. Treating autistic children, or those with ADD, ADHD, or violent behavior problems with drugs that further damage their system is not the answer. It has been proven that the bacterial profile of autistic children is dramatically different from that of healthy children. Pain medications like ibuprofen taken for long periods of time can eventually burn holes in the gut. Teenagers who take antibiotics for acne can eventually alter or destroy enough good bacteria that they develop inflammatory bowel problems and colitis.

For several years, I discounted all the mounting research about the benefits of fermented foods and drinks. Part of my hesitation is that the nurse in me was a germ freak. I never believed in such a thing as "good bacteria." I don't like milk or yogurt. But one taste of Kombucha changed everything. Then I tried fermented vegetables, specifically sauerkraut and beet kvass. I honestly felt so amazing that I include these foods and Kombucha every day. I feel rested and don't crave carbohydrates. They make me feel good, and happy.

I recently found an awesome book by Donna Schwenk, *Cultured Food for Life*. I highly recommend it, as well as her website (see end of chapter for link), with free videos to help you make your own fermented foods and drinks. Donna is so passionate about fermented foods and drinks, and so willing to freely share her story and years of experience, that you will be excited to try a recipe or two. Most people have no idea how absolutely amazing they can feel when they help build good gut flora. Kombucha is loaded with B vitamins and is a powerful detoxifier that flushes heavy metals. Donna was able to reverse high blood pressure and type 2 diabetes herself and has heard from thousands of people over the years about the personal health challenges they have healed. These foods have been around for thousands of years—but now they are becoming popular once again, because even medical research supports the results.

Donna recommends starting slowly with just one half cup of kefir; or four ounces of Kombucha; or a tablespoon or two of fermented vegetables with a meal. Kombucha is becoming a popular replacement for soda and is great for kids too. Always remember to start slowly, with grace, and allow your body to experience vibrant health, abundant energy, and a feeling of peace and happiness. That's my wish for you.

## RESOURCES:

*Integrative Gastroenterology* by Gerard E. Mullin MD.
http://thefoodmd.com/integrative-gastroenterology

*The Second Brain* by Michael Gershon MD.
http://www.harpercollins.com/9780060930721/the-second-brain

*Gut and Psychology Syndrome* by Dr. N. Campbell-McBride.
http://www.doctor-natasha.com/gaps-book.php

*Cultured Foods for Life* by Donna Schwenk may be ordered on her website which is a treasure trove of information! Donna taught me so much about healthy gut bacteria!
http://www.culturedfoodlife.com/

## chapter fourteen

# Juicing with Jay Kordich—
# The "Juiceman" Answers

*Pull out the poison, feed the body, and God will heal.*
—Burton Goldberg

This is really the bottom line to healing at the cellular level. The secret to true healing lies in two places—first in the mind and second in the gut. You *must* address both. I will repeat this: the best food, the strongest pill, stapling or banding your stomach, chemotherapy, radiation, the latest diet craze, advice from Dr. Oz, etc. will not work if you don't work through the underlying emotional issues that are causing you stress. This is one of the biggest differences between Western medicine and naturopathy. When you substitute a pill for a symptom you are adding a poison, not pulling it out.

In order to pull out poison, you have to begin with your mind and toxic thoughts. Most toxic thoughts have to do with our image of who we are told we are. We have to consciously imprint upon our subconscious mind that our true nature is to love and be loved. Dr. Wayne Dyer states it beautifully: "You decide you are a being of divine love, and every time you have a thought that is not consistent with that assessment of who you are, you correct the thought."

How do you correct the thought? You affirm:

» I accept myself unconditionally right now.
» I am divine love.
» All is well.
» Everything is working out for my highest good.
» Out of this situation only good will come.
» I am safe.

These affirmations are from one of my favorite women on the planet, Louise Hay, who started Hay House Publishing at the age of sixty. She is my inspiration and these are from her new book, *All Is Well*. Louise has many amazing books—another one of my favorites is *You Can Heal Your Life*. Her insight into the emotional aspect of physical disease is spot on. I refer to her book with every client.

I never recommend drastic changes all at once unless someone is really seriously committed to that path. So many people won't even consider trying anything outside the Western medicine box because they think they will have to give up all the foods they love. I recommend starting slow and making small yet significant additions to what you eat now.

## Start Where You Are Right Now

If someone tells me I can't have something, it just makes me more determined to find a way to get it! So make small changes with grace and allow your body to heal. Forcing anything just causes resistance, and resistance causes stress.

One of the best things you can do for your health and your body is to begin *adding* fresh organic fruits and vegetables daily. I have been a big fan of Jay Kordich since his famous infomercial days selling the Juiceman Juicer. I loved my Juiceman Juicer and wore out the tape that came with it. I asked Jay about juicing versus blending, and the need for fiber, and he gave me permission to share his information. Jay has dedicated his life to sharing his story of overcoming cancer and of his enormous knowledge of the nutritional benefits of every fruit and vegetable known to man. He has a heart of pure gold.

The following is from Jay Kordich and is used with permission.

"Fiber has zero nutrients in it. It's necessary to *eat* fiber when you are eating foods such as salads, etc. Our mouths have powerful enzymes in them that are designed to help digest foods we chew before we swallow. Once the foods go into our stomach, the digestion starts by separating the juices from the foods we chewed from the fiber. The fiber is excreted through our feces and the juices are absorbed through our bloodstream so we can assimilate the nutrients. This is the *best* way we can use fiber. It's the most natural way. When we blend foods, it does not allow our bodies to use these enzymes in our mouth because we are swallowing quickly, and secondly the intense speed from blenders kill many of the natural enzymes from the friction (speed). And thirdly, we absorb nutrients so much more efficiently when we are juicing versus blending. If you are swallowing the blended foods, your body still has to work hard to separate the fibers from the juices, and it has to do it now without the benefit of the chewing (from your mouth's enzymes that are excreted when you eat). I hope this is clear to you. Now, with all of this being said, I *do* blend foods at least a few times a week with our slow blender. We blend super-foods that can't be juiced and some foods that can't be juiced, like avocados and bananas. In other words, you have to blend soft foods like avocados and bananas. But our powerhouse of nutrients *always* comes from juicing.

"Today I am going to explain what the late, great master teachers (Dr. Max Gerson, Dr. Norman Walker, and Dr. Kirschner) taught to me about the differences between juicing and blending back between 1948 and 1960.

"There are two distinct reasons behind the differences between juicing and blending, but first let's talk about how juicers work and the reasons behind juicing. Some juicers extract the pulp out the back (like our slow juicer The Power Grind Pro does), and other juicers squeeze out the pulp from an auger type of a juicer like the Champion, the Greenstar, the Samson, or the Omega. For example, when you are juicing your greens, the greens hit the blades, and within half a turn it's in your glass, and the pulp is out in the bucket within an instant, so the oxidation process is not as near as intense. However, not all juicers are equal in this aspect. Some juicers spin so fast (16,000 rpms) that the friction is quite high when the produce is hitting the blades. It depends, but it is still by far less aggressive than blending your foods. Juicing extracts all fiber (pulp) from the foods, so that when you are drinking the juice, it's 100 percent free of pulp. Some people think this is not as smart as blending so that all the pulp and juice are combined. This assumption cannot be further from the truth, so this is why I am going to explain it in depth so that you, in turn, can help people understand the truth.

"When you juice fruits/vegetables/seeds/nuts/grains ... whatever it is you are juicing, these *juices* become predigested, meaning they go into our bloodstreams immediately, bypassing any need for digestion because they are in pure juice form. Have you ever drank alcohol and/or coffee and felt the effects from it within just a few minutes? Well that's because alcohol and/or coffee has no pulp in it and has a powerful effect on the body—negatively of course!

"Almost every human being living now has huge challenges with digesting the foods we eat. It's not really about the digestion as much as it is about the 'absorption' of the foods you are eating. Statistics say that as we age, we absorb 10 percent less every ten years of our life. So that by the time we reach the age of fifty, we are only absorbing 50 percent of the foods (nutrients) we are eating and by the time we are eighty years old, we are only absorbing the nutrients from the foods at the rate of 20 percent. Some people absorb only 5-10 percent by the time they reach this age.

"This is why juicing is so important. Absorbing 100 percent of the nutrients is why juicing is an incredible way to feed our bodies. Yet I can understand why so many of us are blending our greens and fruits because it seems natural to say, 'The juice and the fiber are better to consume together, because all this fiber is going to be wasted unless I blend them together.'

"This is not accurate. Let me explain. Yes, juicing is devoid of fiber! Fiber has no nutrients in it, once the juices have been extracted. Fiber that is left behind in your juicer should be used in your compost bin or best used as mulch for your flowerbeds. It should *not* be consumed in the ways we are consuming it through the process of blending.

"However, fiber is quite important … but *only* when fiber is found in the foods you eat, not in foods you are blending. For example, let's say you eat a salad. You begin chewing, and once you start to chew, your salivary glands start to produce enzymes called ptyalin, and another enzyme called amylase. These enzymes secrete saliva so that your foods are absorbed into your stomach easier. As you chew, you swallow. Did you know that the stomach has something called a peristaltic wave? It moves at twenty-two beats per minute, helping us evacuate the fiber from our bodies. Now, once the food is in the stomach, the stomach begins to separate the pulp from the juice. The juice (or liquid) from the salad now is being absorbed through the intestines, when then go into your portal vein, and then into the liver to feed our sixty trillion cells. Meanwhile, the fiber is being pushed through the intestines (which is thirty-three feet combined from the mouth to the anus). This is the reason why we as humans *need* fiber, but through eating our foods. Through this process, the body is doing what a juicer is actually doing, separating the fiber from the juices, so that our bodies can assimilate the nutrients that have been extracted from the fibers. This is why I have been saying for sixty-three years: it's the juice from the fibers that feed you!

"Your juicer is separating the fiber from the pulp so your body can absorb the liquid part of the foods through your intestines and the fiber is being evacuated out of your large bowel, so that, once it is out of the body, it has done its job.

"Blending is quite different. There are two major actions that we need to be aware of before we start to think about blending foods. First, the intense speed factor needs to be considered, and secondly, drinking the juice with the fiber is not a wise choice. I will discuss both of these.

"Number one is digestion. For example, if you are adding green foods such as spinach, kale, parsley, and apples to the water in the blender, we need to realize that adding water to the foods is creating a real challenge to our digestive tract. First, we are not allowing the salivary glands to mix in with the blended foods, so once we swallow it, it has now left our mouth and is sitting in the stomach, but without the proper enzymes to help with digestion! Now the stomach has to begin the process of separating the pulp from the fibers, so that the body can evacuate the pulp out of our body, so that the body can absorb the liquid part of the blended foods. *This* is the process of digestion.

"Did you know that if, even the size of a microscopic fiber were to reach your bloodstream, you would die of a blood clot? This is why the body has to separate the fibers from the juices. Consuming blended juices this way, without the help of the salivary glands, can and most likely causes distension in the stomach, intestinal gas and bloating, and gives us an unnatural feeling of being too full. Plus you will not feel energized, you will feel sleepy because now the blood that was in your head has to go down into the stomach to help digest the blended foods.

"Number two is high speed. The foods you are blending are spinning at unimaginable speeds. Twenty-five thousand revolutions per minute. But it's worse than that. It's really twenty-five thousand times four blades as they spin in unison, or sometimes these newer blenders have six or eight blades. When you multiply those blades times twenty-five thousand ... you get way into the hundred thousand or one hundred fifty thousand revolutions per *minute*. These speeds heat up your foods, destroying the life force as they unnaturally rip apart these tender tissues from the plant's leaves.

"What happens to the food when it's being blended that quickly? Friction and heat is what happens! Through this process, we lose all valuable enzymes that were once in the greens or fruits or foods. We also lose valuable nutrients.

"Why? Because high speed kills enzymes and nutrients and oxidation occurs. This is why *slow* juicers (like our new Power Grind pro) are being designed and manufactured so that, through slower speeds we are preserving the nutrients and the friction is minimal, if not, nonexistent. Now the enzymes we are searching for, and also the powerful antioxidants, phytonutrients, vitamins, and minerals are being preserved, and are intact, ready to be absorbed into your bloodstream, in perfect order.

"This is why I can't understand why people will go to the trouble of purchasing a very expensive slow juicer yet also have a high speed blender. I want to make sure we are looking at these important issues, because as a teacher, this is my job! It's my job to help us all better understand the choices we make to help us build powerful and effective *living kitchens*.

"High speeds kill, so keep your blending to a minimum. Foods such as bananas, avocados, figs, salad dressings, living soups (not cooked), and 99 percent-water fruits such as mangos are great for blending, but just remember that when you are blending, you should have a slower speed blender as you blend your living soups, otherwise they could be called cooked soups! Start your blender off slowly and do not use the high-speed button. This is what [my wife] Linda and I do. For example, we blend about twice a week, but we juice twice a day.

"This is why juicing is entirely different from blending."

Jay and his beautiful wife, Linda, share their knowledge and hundreds of juicing combinations on Facebook and their website: www.jaykordich.com

Jay also has several books that provide both recipes and amazing amounts of information to get you juicing—see his website.

Thank you, Jay!

## chapter fifteen

# Breast Cancer—Pink Ribbons and Tears are Not Enough

In 1974, First Lady Betty Ford publicly announced that she had undergone a mastectomy. This helped to de-stigmatize and bring awareness to a very private and painful issue that many women faced alone. Since that announcement, billions of dollars have been raised in the name of "breast cancer awareness," and to support breast cancer research—but seriously—are we *really* any more aware?

Before you get defensive, close your mind, or start backing away—a reaction I get every time someone asks why I don't support marches and pink ribbons—just for a brief moment please read with an open mind. First, ask yourself a few questions:

» Does the word cancer scare you?
» Before the breast cancer awareness movement, there were essentially three options for treatment: surgery, radiation, and chemotherapy. What current cutting-edge treatments are you aware of today?

» How many of your friends, relatives, and loved ones actually beat cancer after just one of any of the above treatments, only to have it come back somewhere else? How many died?

» How does buying a pink bucket of fried chicken or a pink beer pong table empower you to seek true research?

» Here's my last and most important question: Where does the money you raise at any of the marches go? I am not talking about "it goes to the state march-for-life office." Where do each of those dollars go, and how does it help women get cutting-edge treatment and the latest research? That is the purpose, right?

No one has ever been able to trace the money for me, from the hard-earned and hard-fought battles on high school tracks all over America to the end of the money trail.

The first use of a pink ribbon in connection with breast cancer awareness was when the Susan G. Komen Foundation handed them out to participants in its New York City race for breast cancer survivors in 1991. The following year, the pink ribbon was adopted as the official symbol of National Breast Cancer Awareness Month. Alexandra Penney, the editor in chief of *Self* magazine, and Evelyn Lauder, the senior corporate vice president of Estee Lauder Cosmetics Company, and a breast cancer survivor herself, created the ribbon for distribution to stores and businesses in New York City.

However, the first breast cancer ribbon was actually peach colored and created by a much lesser-known sixty-eight-year-old woman named Charlotte Haley in 1990. Charlotte was a breast cancer survivor along with four generations of her family that had also fought the disease. Charlotte made the ribbons by hand at her own dining room table and personally handed them out with a card attached, which read, "The National Cancer Institute's annual budget is 1.8 billion US dollars, and only 5 percent goes to cancer prevention. Help us wake up our legislators and America by wearing this ribbon."

Charlotte distributed thousands of these cards and ribbons by hand and in addition, wrote to many prominent women (such as former first ladies and Abigail van Buren of "Dear Abby" fame) to enlist their help in spreading the word about breast cancer *prevention.*

In 1992, the year after the huge success of the pink ribbon giveaway, Alexandra Penney and Evelyn Lauder approached Charlotte Haley to attempt to adapt her idea with theirs and work together. Charlotte soundly rejected their offer and refused to be part of what she felt was a commercial effort. Ribbons were big business—after all, the *New York Times* declared 1992 "The Year of the Ribbon"—but Lauder and *Self* magazine were not to be dissuaded. High-powered lawyers came up with answer: change the color of the ribbon. They chose "150 pink"—one of their most popular colors. In the fall of 1992, Estee Lauder collected more than 200,000 pink ribbon petitions, urging the White House to push for increased funding for breast cancer research. The peach ribbon and Charlotte Haley were history.

Meanwhile, another national movement was gaining ground. National Breast Cancer Awareness Month was founded and initiated by a British chemical company called Imperial Chemical Industries (ICI) in 1985. This was in partnership with the American Cancer Society and the pharmaceutical division of ICI, Zeneca. Imperial Chemical Industries manufactures and sells pesticides, plastics, and pharmaceuticals. Its chemical plant in Ohio was identified in 1996 as the *third-largest source of cancer-causing pollution in the United States.*

The American subsidiary of ICI is AstraZeneca. In 1997, after the acquisition of a chain of cancer treatment centers, Zeneca merged with a Swedish pharmaceutical company called Astra to form AstraZeneca, *creating the world's third-largest pharmaceutical entity.*

AstraZeneca manufactures one of the world's top-selling breast cancer drugs, tamoxifen. In 1998, The National Cancer Institute hailed tamoxifen as "preventing" breast cancer when taken continuously (usually for a period of five years), despite the fact that known side effects were serious blood clots in the legs and lungs and increased risk of cancer elsewhere, such as endometrial and uterine. Additionally, in 2009, a study published in the journal *Cancer Research* found that *long-term tamoxifen use increased the risk of an aggressive, difficult-to-treat estrogen receptor negative second cancer in the opposite breast.* The National Cancer Institute provided funding for the research. Did they stop prescribing tamoxifen? No.

One of the only attempts at "prevention" was the promotion of yearly mammograms—with slogans like "Early detection is your best prevention." Unfortunately, by the time cancer shows up on a mammogram, it is far too late to "prevent" it. Additionally—it has finally been acknowledged that radiation exposure from yearly routine mammography may actually *cause* more cases of breast cancer than it identifies in younger women. Squeezing breasts between two metal plates has also been shown to damage delicate lymph tissue, causing it to rupture. The National Cancer Institute reports that mammograms misidentify tumors some percentage of the time, resulting in additional invasive and unnecessary procedures, and causing needless anxiety.

Radiation in the form of mammography or treatment seems counterintuitive to the prevention or elimination of cancer. Why is it that we are told to avoid and protect ourselves from harmful X-rays (dental for example) that could cause cancer, and then we turn around and treat cancer with the same harmful radiation? Why do we allow our breasts to be squeezed between two metal plates that expose us to the equivalent of forty chest X-rays and run the risk of rupturing a harmless cyst or tumor? Two CT head scans are enough radiation to cause a genetic mutation, and the risk of soft-tissue sarcoma doubles. Radiation does not prevent or cure cancer. Neither does chemically poisoning the body with chemotherapy.

Chemotherapy and radiation remove tumors. Tumors are clusters of cancer cells. Once destroyed, where do these cells go? They go into the bloodstream to be eliminated. Chemotherapy, radiation and even surgery do not treat the circulating cancer cells. You must get rid of these cells in the blood to be truly free of cancer. The way to eliminate these cells is with detoxification (pull out the poisons) and then to feed the body essential minerals and nutrients to build healthy red blood cells and bone marrow. In order for you to be healed of cancer, it must be completely gone from both scans and your blood. Western medicine measures the amount of circulating tumor cells in your blood by a blood test for "cancer markers."

A German doctor and cancer survivor, Dr. Ryke Geerd Hamer, did an enormous amount of research about the emotional aspect of cancer. His research is extremely scientific and undeniably proves that most cancers are related to an unresolved emotional conflict. Here are the emotional precursors to the breast cancer issues:

Breast Milk Gland: Involving Care or Disharmony
Breast Mild Duct: Separation Conflict
Breast Left: Conflict concerning Child, Home or Mother
Breast Right: Conflict with Partner or Others

If you don't first deal with the emotional work, you won't heal. This lesson is repeated until it is learned. With breast cancer, the emotional issue is all about relationships, nurturing, mothering, and nourishment. Breasts represent nourishment. At our mother's breast, we are given life. At the deepest, cellular level, breast issues represent a refusal to nourish the self. Did you lose your mother? Do you feel you put everyone else first? Does your partner nourish your need to be loved—deeply, unconditionally—and even more importantly, do you *feel* that love? Is your partner faithful? Women are intuitive. They know. Women want to please—many times denying their own needs—the deepest of which is to be wanted, appreciated, needed, and loved.

Cutting off your breasts does not guarantee you will never get cancer. If you remove part or all of a cancerous lung yet continue to smoke, you have not removed the probable cause. The best way to prevent any cancer is to make changes to your lifestyle—slowly, and with grace so these changes become good habits. Genetics alone does not predispose you to a certain disease. Epigenetics (the study of the way in which the expression of heritable traits is modified by environmental influences or other mechanisms without a change to the DNA sequence) is proving that lifestyle is a far more accurate indicator of cancer probability. Many reproductive cancers are found during periods of great hormonal change—breast cancers found during pregnancy; ovarian and uterine cancers found at menopause. In many cases, the use of artificial estrogens taken for years (such as birth control pills and hormone replacement therapy) precede the diagnosis. The human body cannot process chemical estrogens and stores them in estrogen-receptive tissues like lymph and breast tissue. If not eliminated, these cells form cysts and tumors. Of course the diagnosis of cancer at any time is a multifaceted issue, and the best we can do is share knowledge of successful treatments and empower each other. There is no place for paralyzing fear, guilt, or self-doubt that allows us to make decisions that appear to be our only choice in the present—with great consequence in the future. Epigenetics is proving that living holistically—with conscious lifestyle and food choice; conscious affirmations, thoughts and beliefs; detox from artificial steroidal hormones; thermography instead of mammograms; deep breathing; a little sunshine and exercise; and most of all, love for yourself and everyone—has a greater effect on our health and longevity than our genetics. The best research is that which is done with your own eyes, ears, intuition, and open mind. Find your truth—not my truth expressed here, but your truth. Do your own research. My hope is to educate, empower, and inspire you to push past paralyzing fear, to enable you to make decisions from a place of love.

Here are two very moving, poignant examples of real women and the truth about early detection and breast cancer.

The Scar Project by photographer David Jay is a beautiful and moving series of large-scale portraits of young (ages eighteen to thirty-five) breast-cancer survivors from all over the world. "The Scar Project is an exercise in awareness, hope, reflection, and healing. The mission is three-fold: raise public consciousness of early-onset breast cancer, raise funds for breast cancer research/ outreach programs and help young survivors see their scars, faces, figures, and experiences through a new, honest, and ultimately empowering lens." David Jay

The Promise—a documentary exposing the truth about breast cancer.

## RESOURCES:

http://www.thescarproject.org

http://www.nbcam.org

http://www.astrazeneca.com/Home

http://www.cancer.gov/cancertopics/factsheet/Therapy/hormone-therapy-breast

http://www.whale.to/cancer/breast6.html

http://www.preventcancer.com/about/epstein.htm

http://www.bcaction.org/2012/03/08/charlotte-didnt-sell-out-neither-should-we

http://thinkbeforeyoupink.org/?page_id=26

http://www.alternative-cancer-care.com/dr-ryke-geerd-hamer.html

http://thepromisefilm.net

## chapter sixteen

# Lyme Disease—Appreciating the Stealthy Spirochete

*In order to successfully treat organisms as complex and as highly intelligent as the mycoplasmas, it is important to first get rid of all sense you may have of superiority to "stupid" bacteria due to our "superior" intelligence. Second, it is crucial to understand what they do and why they do it—and to begin to intervene in that process in a sophisticated way, that is, for us to adapt our own behaviors to theirs. In other words, to be like Ginger Rogers in relation to Fred Astaire—doing everything he did but in high heels and backward. And with respect for their capacities, to begin to intervene in what they do at the subtlest levels possible.*
—Stephen Harrod Buhner

I love being outside. In fact, if it's a sunny day—no matter the temp—I *have* to get out. My peace is sometimes ruined, however, by stinkbugs, and I do worry about ticks as I walk in the woods or on trails. Be sure to check yourself, your kids, and your pets for ticks. Lyme disease is the most widespread vector-borne disease in the United States.

"Harvard researchers estimate there are nearly two hundred fifty thousand new Lyme disease infections—only 10 percent of which will be accurately diagnosed" (from *Healing Lyme Disease*

*Coinfections* by Stephen Harrod Buhner). Stephen is an amazing herbalist and this book—as well as his first book, *Healing Lyme*—is the most comprehensive, cutting-edge, well-researched information you will find. If you want to know more, or know someone struggling with Lyme disease, please share this blog and all the links to valuable information, protocols, herbs, and resources. I love all of Stephen's books, and his writing style is so well researched yet entertaining.

The absolutely best method for treating Lyme disease is the same as any other—and that is *prevention*. Check your body frequently if you have been outdoors in any area where ticks could crawl or fall on you. This applies to your head and hair as well, so as soon as possible check your entire body and *be thorough*. At this early stage, they probably aren't attached to you yet. There are some exceptions—but generally speaking, an infected tick must be attached to your skin for twenty-four hours to transmit the Lyme bacteria— which are, in actuality, the toxic excretion from the infecting vector (the tick) that must first enjoy a lovely blood meal from the host (that would be you).

(A lovely Chianti with that, perhaps?)

The blood from the host must travel to the tick's stomach. While there, the Lyme spirochetes determine what kind of animal the tick is feeding on and immediately begin to alter their outer protein structure (coat) to enable them to live unnoticed in that particular host.

Lyme disease is not a virus. It is a spirochete parasite. According to Buhner, there are what he calls "*coinfective* bacteria" that interact in both the vector that spreads them and the host that receives them. These bacteria are some of the most "potent, resistant bacterial organisms" known to man.

Therefore, taking a single treatment, a one-therapy approach that was formulated in the nineteenth century and based on identifying a single bacteria and killing it with an antibiotic is rather archaic, wouldn't you agree? These bacteria belong to the same band of brothers as salmonella, pseudomonas, E. coli, cholera, gonorrhea, and helicobacter, and they have shared survival and antibiotic resistance strategies over dinner and know how to win. These bacteria are highly evolved after years of antibiotic resistance and adaptation.

So don't invite them to dinner.

Perhaps if we understand how these *specific* bacteria outsmart our overburdened immune system, we can develop treatment plans for each individual and address the specific symptoms that are destroying their quality of life. Lyme disease is devastating because it can affect joints, organs, and even the brain.

Here's why. When these bacteria are ingested by ticks, they immediately infect the *epithelial cells* of their GI tract and begin traveling to the insects salivary glands, where they are then injected into human (mammal) bloodstreams by the bite of the tick. The metamorphosis these vector-borne bacteria undergo immediately gives us some idea of how incredibly adaptable and resilient they are. Human (mammal) blood is completely different from an insect's stomach.

Insects do not have hemoglobin, they have *hemolymph,* which does not carry oxygen because insects breathe (respirate) from their body surfaces. Mammal blood has a *higher pH* than an insect's stomach. So in literally a few seconds, these bacteria go from a low-oxygen, low-temp, low-pH stomach to a completely opposite bloodstream. Instantly they have the ability to analyze their new environment and initiate the necessary changes in their physiology to survive in their new home.

You have to appreciate their intelligence and adaptability.

And it goes without saying—but you know I *have* to say it anyway—if your well-loved and cared-for body is alive with richly *oxygenated* and beautifully balanced highly alkaline *pH blood,* the dinner party will end sooner and these warriors can return to their real home in the ecosystem. Spirochete bacteria become a major problem when your immune system is compromised from lack of self-care, stress, poor dietary choices, etc. The more depressed the immune system, the worse the symptoms.

**Hematopoietic stem cells** (HSCs) are the blood cells that differentiate into all the other blood cells. They are created in the bone marrow. They flow throughout the entire body in the bloodstream. They differentiate into endothelial cells, red blood cells, T cells, platelets, etc. The Lyme spirochetes have a very strong affinity for endothelial cells and red blood cells. They must have both of them to survive. They are also rather fond of collagen tissue. Endothelial cells line all the blood vessels and their cavities in your body, the surfaces of your glands, the interior surfaces of the heart (the endocardium), all the lymphatic capillaries, and are present in the liver, spine, and bone marrow.

Once the spirochetes have entered the bloodstream, they double in number every twenty-four hours and begin to colonize or "seed" four sites immediately: the red blood cells, the spleen, the liver, and the bone marrow. Initially, a person may not show any symptoms. When the acute symptoms do occur they are flu-like: fatigue, general malaise, and fever. These symptoms may last for several weeks until the bacterial count drops dramatically. "Early in the infectious stage, large numbers of bacteria are created and released into the blood. But this peaks between ten and fourteen days post-infection and thereafter begins to decrease." (Buhner from *Healing Lyme Disease Coinfections* 2013). When the initial symptoms go away, some people think they have eliminated the bacteria. However, most people are, in truth, an asymptomatic *carrier.*

After the initial infectious phase and the spirochetes are firmly established in the body, they rapidly begin to spread. "Approximately every five days they release new bacteria into the blood. Every colonized site in the body will release new organisms *simultaneously.* Studies have shown that the organisms that are released into the bloodstream during these intervals tend to be genetically different each time. In other words, the bacteria are developing unique strains every five days in order to avoid an effective immune response" (Buhner).

**This is a long-term, sustained, multi-location parasite attack.** This is what makes these bacteria so difficult to deal with and eliminate. Lyme spirochetes need nutrients and minerals that they obtain from collagen tissue, endothelial cells, bone marrow, and hemoglobin—and they attack and feed upon these areas and then deplete your body of vital nutrients. They replicate at random times and in multiple locations simultaneously—which makes it difficult for your immune system to react quickly enough. This is also why the symptoms vary so dramatically that they are often misdiagnosed. If the spirochetes feed off the collagen tissue in your knee, you have Lyme arthritis; if they feed off the endothelial tissue in your heart, you have bacterial endocarditis; if they feed off endothelial cells in your brain, the infection in your brain will cause meningitis or encephalitis. The best defense is a great offense. If your immune system is healthy and you actively put good bacteria in your gut, as well as pull out the bad bacteria from your blood as soon as possible—before the spirochetes set up camp in their favorite feeding grounds—you have a much better chance of minimizing their spread and ultimately cause their demise.

Many physicians look at the symptoms and try to match them to some type of predetermined protocol. They also tend to rely upon pharmaceutical treatment and antibiotics, and when the symptoms disappear, believe the disease to be healed. One of the most important factors in treating these super-bacterial infections is a strong, healthy immune system. Your body knows perfectly and exactly how to heal itself.

The goal for treatment then is to first prevent the tick from attaching itself to you. Check your whole body for ticks as soon as possible if you have been outdoors and think you might have been around tick-friendly areas. Make sure, *if you send your kids to summer camp*, or if their grandparents or someone other than you are picking them up after outdoor activities—your children know to check themselves for ticks, or ask someone to help them check. If you find a tick attached, the first thing to do is remove the tick and try to draw out the bacteria from the bite site as soon as possible within the first twenty-four hours of the initial bite. Once you draw out the bacteria, you need to alkalize the blood and at the same time, kill any circulating bacteria that escaped the bite site. Remember, with bacteria, it is always a matter of numbers. The sooner you destroy and eliminate the infecting organisms, the less likely it is they will travel to feeding sites throughout your body and set up colonies. Ingesting healthy bacteria that form large colonies that crowd out the bad may be helpful too.

Buhner appropriately says, "The bacteria are evolving. We should, too."


## RESOURCES:

http://buhnerhealinglyme.com/bookstore

# chapter seventeen

# You Put the Lyme in the Bentonite—a Natural Healing Approach

*You have your way. I have my way. As for the right way,*
*the correct way, and the only way, it does not exist.*
—Friedrich Nietzsche

If by chance you find a tick embedded in your skin, remove it as soon as possible. The best way is to grasp it firmly with pointy tweezers and pull straight up. (See a link at the end of this chapter for a video demonstrating tick removal.)

Immediately after removing the tick, cover the area with a paste made from water and bentonite clay. This clay has the ability to instantly draw out the poisonous bacteria. Bentonite clay can adsorb many times its weight and hold the toxins taken in until your body can eliminate them. So by using it topically, you can draw out toxins from the skin, and by taking it internally, you can draw out toxins from within. This clay has many uses and is great for immediate relief of acid indigestion as well—it has a pH of 8-plus. Along with the clay, after drawing out the toxins, immediately spray the skin with colloidal silver. Colloidal silver was very popular before antibiotics. Colloidal silver is safe and effective against many bacteria including MRSA and is a powerful anti-inflammatory. It also can be applied topically immediately following the clay, and then taken internally if desired. Remember, if you can draw out the bacteria as soon as you find the tick, or at least within twenty-four hours, you have a very good chance of eliminating the bacteria before they have a chance to multiply and colonize.

I just want to remind you that I never recommend anything I haven't personally used myself or wouldn't feel safe giving my own children. I only buy products from trusted sources—there are many others from which to chose—but these are my personal choice. Please know I do not receive compensation for any products I suggest.

Charconite is a brilliant product from Markus Rothkranz combining two of the most powerful natural substances for pulling toxins, bacteria, etc. out of your body. Taken internally, it will detoxify your blood. Charcoal has been used for years to reverse medical overdose, drug and alcohol overdose, and food poisoning. Charcoal tablets absorb everything and get it out. You can also take activated charcoal that is available at most grocery and drug stores and online.

I personally keep all three of these products (bentonite clay, colloidal silver, and charcoal) on hand. They are great to have for many issues—from acne breakouts to bug bites to poison ivy to indigestion—you will find many uses.

Sometime in the 1500s, during the European Renaissance, a master physician, alchemist, astronomer, and herbalist named Paracelsus made popular a theory he called the "doctrine of signatures." He and many other herbalists believed that every plant was given a "signature," and the shape, color, texture, taste, and habitat of the plant were a clue to its healing properties. For example, kidney beans are shaped like kidneys, walnuts look like the human brain, and Hawaiians regard the banana as a symbol of male fertility or "comfort with their maleness."

## Hang Loose, Brudda

The first case of Lyme disease occurred in Lyme, Connecticut. According to the Invasive Plant Atlas of New England, the Japanese knotweed plant populates many areas of the world, but the most concentrated growth occurs in areas where there is a high infestation of the Lyme bacteria *Borrelia*. Knotweed is native to Japan and other Asian countries and was brought to the United States for decorative and ornamental reasons, but it is now despised because it is invasive and suffocates all other plants nearby.

Japanese knotweed grows rampantly in Lyme, Connecticut.

## Where There Is Disease You Will Also Find Treatment

If Lyme disease becomes chronic, the spirochetes travel to and colonize in many areas of the body; Japanese knotweed herbal supplements are antibacterial and have the ability to cross the blood-brain barrier and safely and effectively bind toxins. The supplements have become increasingly popular as potent antioxidants, cardiovascular system tonics, anti-aging tonics, and for the treatment of Lyme disease and Lyme-related arthritis. It is suggested to use the whole root of the herb—benefits may be seen within two weeks to two months. Work with a knowledgeable herbalist as far as dose and length of treatment.

Paracelsus probably never heard of "resveratrol," and you may not have either—but amazing studies have been conducted into the anti-aging, Alzheimer's treating, cancer-preventative, and longevity-enhancing properties of this substance—*wow*—just to name a few! The knotweed plant is the greatest source of resveratrol, and there are indications that resveratrol influences many genetic pathways, which may explain its ability to lengthen life. In the current epigenetic studies of longevity, resveratrol is number one! Most resveratrol supplements sold in the United States are extracted from the knotweed plant.

There are other herbs (in addition to knotweed) that work on specific organs or areas affected. Buhner's website has several sources for purchasing these and also additional information that is not in his book. (See resources page at end of this chapter.)

## Herbs for Chronic Issues

- » Hawthorn—my favorite for heart issues
- » Milk thistle—the best for liver issues; can even reverse cirrhosis
- » Cat's claw—anti-inflammatory and anti-spirochete
- » Sarsaparilla—good for liver, grows where Lyme is most prevalent
- » Rhodiola—one of Buhner's favorites: "It is specific for chronic, long-term fatigue, recurrent infections, recovery from long-term illness and infections, nervous exhaustion, chronic fatigue syndrome, chronic disease conditions with depression, low immune function, brain fog, acceleration of recovery from debilitating conditions."

With bacteria, it is always a matter of numbers. Good bacteria found in kefir, Kombucha, and fermented vegetables put fifty or more strains of good, healthy bacteria in your gut. Good yeast used to be used by hospitals to treat bad yeast. Coconut kefir, for example, kills candida. Kimchi kills bird flu and heals the bird.

Remember, if you live in areas where Lyme disease has been found, the best defense is to be proactive and boost your immune system before tick season, and to check your body very carefully after you have been outside. Please be sure to educate your children about this too. Many times kids are away at summer camps for a week or more or they spend time away from home, and they need to check daily for ticks. It is so much easier to prevent Lyme disease than to diagnose and treat it. Bacteria are intelligent. Respect them.

## RESOURCES:

http://www.1stchineseherbs.com/lyme_disease.html

http://bodyecology.com/

http://buhnerhealinglyme.com/bookstore

http://www.culturedfoodlife.com/

http://markusrothkranz.com/online-store/bodyforce/charconite.html

Tick removal:
www.youtube.com/watch?v=0wotB38WrRY&feature=youtu.be

Fermented Foods:
http://www.culturedfoodlife.com

http://www.chelseagreen.com/content/the-art-of-fermentation-is-now-a-new-york-times-bestseller

http://search.longevitywarehouse.com/search?Search=coconut+kefir

## chapter eighteen

# Resistance Is Futile—
# Living with Chronic Disease
# Is not Vital Energy

Time and time again my friends have told me they gave someone with so-called "incurable" cancer, diabetes, or some other chronic illness my e-mail or phone number. I am so grateful—always—for their continued trust in me.

But many times the people never call. Perhaps due to fear or lack of knowledge—perhaps they have no idea what a naturopath does, or perhaps they think they are going to have to eat tofu and meditate for hours and give up all the food they love.

Nothing could be further from the truth.

Why else would someone dependent upon an insulin pump or an oxygen tank or thirty pills a day for survival not at least be willing to try to work with their body to regain vital energy and true healing? Any time you work *against your innate natural healing ability* you are creating *resistance,* and that is an exercise in futility. This applies to diet, medication, surgery, business, money, etc.

And unless you are *truly* sick and tired of being sick and tired—or depressed, or obese, or diabetic, or always short of breath—and you *choose* to completely change your lifestyle, *forcing* drastic change upon a person is temporary and creates the "quick fix" attitude of Western medicine: "How long do I have to drink this fresh juice before I can go back to diet soda?" Or people think they can substitute an herb for a blood-pressure pill and continue to live the same stress-filled life and get different results.

Nothing could be further from the truth.

I find these words of wisdom by John Ramsey (www.TargetingExcellence.com) inspiring:

> One of the biggest traps we fall into is forcing *change*, such as trying to discipline ourselves and saying to ourselves, "I have to do this." "I have to lose weight." "I have to work harder." That very push is the subconscious working against the end result. Any time you tell yourself you "have to" do something, it is the job of your subconscious to say, "No, you don't. You don't have to do anything. I'll get you out of it." And with creative avoidance, procrastination, or in any way possible, you find a way not to do it. When you say, "I have to," you are saying "I have to, but if I had my own way, I would rather be doing something else." The harder you try to do something, the more you work against your natural subconscious creative mechanism.
>
> When I recognize I can, I choose to, or I want to change because it is my idea to become like that, then I have a power inside me that most people have chosen to give up. Once I recognize I am a self-made person both in success and failure and that this success or failure is mine to control, I will stop saying "I have to," and instead say "I *choose* to." I can be as my image tells me I can and move constructively toward that end result with an exciting, magnetic energy and drive that expects excellence!

The exact second you tell yourself, I *can't* have sugar any more—I *can't* eat dairy (*whaat—no ice cream?*)—"Oh, sorry, Grandma dear, I'm fasting this year and *can't* eat your famous 'turducken'"—you create resistance.

Resistance builds muscles. Resistance builds will. But resistance to the natural flow of electromagnetic healing energy builds chronic disease.

Any time you have an experience in your life that is really traumatic, any time you experience intense emotions, those emotions are forever imprinted in your memory. Love, fear, anger, sorrow are all frozen in time in the cells of memory. This has been proven and documented in hundreds of cases of heart donors—where the person receiving the organ feels intense feelings of love for a stranger but turns out to be a person who was loved by the donor.

In one case, an eight-year-old girl received the heart of a ten-year-old girl who had been murdered. The eight-year-old girl began having nightmares about being murdered. After a few sessions with a psychiatrist, the police were notified. The little girl said she knew the man who killed her donor. She was accurately able to describe exactly the time, the weapon, the place, the clothes he wore, and what his victim told him. The police tracked the man down and everything she said was accurate and true. He was convicted on her evidence. Your miraculous heart never forgets—a reason why love is such a powerful, magnetic healing force. Love transcends even death.

When you build resistance in your everyday life—say due to stress, anger, fear, etc.—you create resistance to their opposites. If you cut an electrical wire and put in a carbonized resistor and splice it back together, you change the flow of the current. The source of energy is still there, but it isn't flowing as harmoniously. And so it is with the human body. As resistance builds, the innate life force is *inhibited* and eventually *blocked*. The reason this causes chronic disease is because you are holding it with your thoughts. When you hold contradictions to life, either consciously or unconsciously, you build resistance—which inhibits and blocks your vital energy, or life force. These energy blocks eventually manifest physically as tension headaches, arthritis, high blood pressure, and even cancer.

In many cultures that practice the Eastern philosophy of healing, the human body is viewed as a pathway of meridians, winds, or energy wheels. This vital energy has many names—chi, qi, prana, shakti, life force, etc., depending on the culture.

We become "devitalized" for essentially two reasons—because we don't have enough life force or because these energy channels, or meridians, become "blocked" or "inhibited." In Chinese medicine, it is believed that *stress, toxins*, and *negative emotions* cause blockages in the flow of subtle energy. It is believed that these blockages are the root *cause* of all disturbances or sickness. According to Chinese doctors, all sickness manifests first as an energy blockage before it manifests as a physical disease. You can replenish your prenatal life force, or "jing," by eating more live, photon-rich food (filled with energy from sunlight), and by taking superior or tonic herbs. You can unblock energy meridians in a variety of ways—by the practice of acupuncture, qigong, yoga, etc. In Eastern philosophy, the goal is to work with the body to restore vital energy in order to fulfill your purpose.

Western medicine, with all its technological advances and pharmaceutical wonder drugs, tends to reduce the human body to organs and parts, viruses, bacteria, and cancers—which are diagnosed, isolated, and treated individually—to relieve a *symptom* or group of symptoms. Often times, with the disappearance of symptoms, it is assumed that the treatment was effective, and the person resumes those lifestyle behaviors that caused the disturbance in the first place.

We are electromagnetic beings. Every cell in our magnificent and miraculously created bodies possesses infinite intelligence. Every cell knows perfectly and exactly how to heal the whole because every cell works together. We are not single organs or body parts that can be pulled out of a bag of skin, treated and returned. So anytime you try to isolate a part of the body or a specific organ and *force* some type of synthetic, unnatural therapeutic action upon it—you are creating *resistance*—and all fellow cells and organs will respond accordingly *against* it—to attempt to regain control and bring the whole body back into balance.

Don't get me wrong. All healing has a place; and for acute issues, Western medicine—with all of its technological advances and pharmaceutical wonder drugs—can do miraculous things.

Chronic a.k.a. *lifestyle* issues are another story.

Most doctors are quick to prescribe medication for the treatment of high blood pressure. There are many drugs, but they fall into essentially two categories: *blockers* and *inhibitors*.

There are alpha blockers, beta blockers, calcium channel blockers, and angiotensin inhibitors. All of these drugs artificially lower blood pressure.

Your heart is an engineering miracle. It beats 70 times per minute, 4200 times per hour, 100,800 per day, and 36,720,000 per year. All the blood in the body passes through the heart every three minutes. You essentially move 125 55-gallon barrels of blood each day. Miracle? Yes! Your heart possesses infinite intelligence that allows it to make continual, instant, imperceptible adjustments to rate and strength of contractions in order to keep just enough pressure inside the arterial walls to maintain a harmonious flow of blood.

When your blood pressure drops, the volume of fluid in your blood vessels decreases as well. If you were to lose too much fluid, your blood vessels would collapse and you would die.

I know from personal experience what a horrible feeling it is when your blood pressure drops. After the needle was put in my back for my epidural anesthetic—in prep for my second C-section— my blood pressure dropped to 60/0. I instinctively knew something was wrong, and being a nurse, I asked my husband what the number on the monitor was for my blood pressure. I could literally feel the life draining from my body. It honestly felt like I was falling into a big, silent, white abyss.

Your kidneys are two miraculous bidirectional organs—they can either retain sodium and water (raising blood pressure) or release sodium and water (lowering blood pressure). Your kidneys and heart work together *naturally* to regulate blood pressure fluctuations from exercise, stress, diet, hormone changes, and even severe blood loss.

When you take any pill for high blood pressure, you artificially *force* the blood vessels to dilate, or you artificially block an enzyme in the bloodstream that raises blood pressure. Your perceptive kidneys think you are losing fluid volume, and in an effort to save your life and prevent your arteries from collapsing, your kidneys retain sodium and water—sodium being the electrical conductor you *must* have for heartbeat, brainwave, and muscle health (sodium meaning "Na" on the periodic table of elements, a.k.a. natural salt from the earth, not bleached white table salt).

So now you return to your doctor and your blood pressure is lower, but your legs are filling up with fluid. Any time you *block* or *inhibit* the natural flow of blood, that fluid volume has to go somewhere, and your body knows it must move it away from the heart. So all that water and sodium is retained as far from your heart as possible—in your legs and eventually your hands. Makes sense, right? If you are driving and come to a roadblock, sooner or later traffic will get backed up and have to be diverted around the area.

So your doctor is pleased that your blood pressure is coming down and has a remedy for that fluid buildup—he gives you a diuretic, which *artificially* stimulates your kidneys to release salt and water—that is, instead of storing it—sending it to the bladder. Once it goes to the bladder, there is no going back. If you have ever been on a "water pill," you know how fast this works!

Western medicine substitutes a pill for a function. When you take a blood pressure pill, you substitute artificial regulation for innate intelligence that knows what to do to naturally regulate your blood pressure. When you add a diuretic, you force your kidneys to override their innate intelligence to hold or release water, causing them to resist what they are preprogrammed to do by their Creator without any help from you. Eventually, your body becomes dependent upon artificial regulation, and organs stop functioning.

It's the same thing with insulin. You tell your beloved pancreas, "Don't worry, if I keep shoving sugar and carbohydrates at you by the spoonful, and I sit around all day and don't exercise to move that sugar out of the bloodstream and into my muscles, where it will be utilized as energy instead of stored as fat, there's a pill I can take to fix that. Relax, pancreas, dear. When that stops working, there's a pump or a needle."

So now the kidneys rapidly release this sodium and water from your legs—so rapidly in fact that potassium goes along for the ride—and your muscles begin to *lose fluid volume* and start cramping up, telling you to please pass the potassium or we're going to collapse. Those big white potassium pills are nasty.

And so it is. Because most doctors do not put you on blood pressure medicine with the idea of ever taking you off it, the rest of your life becomes a game of artificial regulation.

And then there are side effects, like dizziness, fatigue, dehydration, impotence in men, depression, and chronic cough. Even if you do eventually find the right combination of blood pressure pill, water pill, and potassium pill—is this really vibrant health? Is impotence and depression something you really want to live with at age thirty-five or forty? High blood pressure isn't just for old people anymore—with increased stress, decreased physical activity, and obesity, even young kids develop it.

In the natural realm, every cell and organ system work together. There are no blockers and inhibitors.

Stress hormones elevate an enzyme called *renin*. Renin is an enzyme released by the kidneys to elevate blood pressure.

Renin-secreting cells are very sensitive to blood flow and fluid loss and are designed to save your life in the event of excess fluid loss from vomiting, diarrhea, and excessive perspiration. As your blood pressure goes up, so does your internal thermostat, and your kidneys then readjust and naturally excrete water via perspiration. If you lose too much water, your kidneys reabsorb water. If you proactively and consciously learn to decrease your stress, you naturally decrease renin levels, which naturally lowers your blood pressure. Slow, deep breathing and meditative practices such as qigong, yoga, and tai chi decrease stress hormones naturally. Exercise and singing bring oxygen to the lungs and heart. Get some sunshine. The best way to heal your heart is to fall in love—and stay there.

When will we ever understand that until you learn to deal with whatever it is that stresses you out, or whatever you eat or drink or think is polluting your bloodstream and blocking your vital energy—that is, *the cause*—until you learn to deal with the cause and work with your body to naturally maintain balance, pills are just a poor substitute. You can't continue to violate the laws of nature and expect to heal. Pills have side effects that create the need for more pills. Nature has no side effects.

No pill or treatment will ever restore your vital energy unless you consciously choose to change your lifestyle and eliminate the cause of the imbalance. We are not meant to live life tethered to an oxygen tank, dependent on pills for mere existence, or canned energy to keep us awake—that is artificially forcing the body to resist what it knows to be unnatural. Resistance causes the body to be at war with itself. Trust instead your innate God-given ability to heal.

## RESOURCES:

http://www.amazon.com/A-Change-Heart-Memoir/dp/0446604690

http://www.britannica.com/EBchecked/topic/498140/renin-angiotensin-system

Sylvia Claire: *A Change of Heart*. An excellent book about organ recipient memories

http://www.amazon.com/A-Change-Heart-Memoir/dp/0446604690

chapter nineteen

# Yes, America, Fukushima Is a *Big* Deal

As more and more information is leaked from the Fukushima radiation disaster site in Japan, the long-term global consequences are impossible to ignore. And yes, America is already experiencing the effects of toxic radiation.

The future of the Fukushima disaster is written in the long-since-forgotten history of Chernobyl. If governments continue to suppress the truth to minimize the damage, withhold vital information from international regulators and knowledgeable scientists, and persecute doctors trying to save children and their parents from the effects of deadly radiation, then the lessons learned and the lives lost will have been in vain. Chernobyl survivors and their offspring suffered and continue to suffer (twenty-five-plus years later) from a wide variety of illnesses due to the exposure to radioactivity in the air, the water, and in the soil, which remains contaminated. The radioactive material in the wastewater from Fukushima that has *already* been discharged into the Pacific Ocean is the largest single amount in history. And it continues to leak daily.

The radiation discharged in the air and sea from these disasters is the toxic imposter of the element *iodine,* a critical trace mineral that your body needs but cannot make. It is the *function* of the thyroid gland to take dietary or supplemental iodine and convert it into the thyroid hormones triiodothyronine (T3) and thyroxine (T4). Thyroid cells are the only cells in the body that can absorb the iodine necessary to make these hormones. Every cell in the human body depends on thyroid hormone to some degree—for normalizing metabolism, for physical and mental development, for balanced mood, regulating healthy blood pressure, preventing adrenal fatigue, boosting immunity, and to maintain the health of our reproductive organs.

One test used to measure thyroid function is called the RAI uptake test. This test measures how much radioactive iodine is "taken up" by the thyroid gland. Cells of the thyroid normally absorb iodine from our bloodstream (obtained from the foods we eat) and use it to make thyroid hormone, which is necessary for many critical bodily functions. The test is administered by giving a dose of radioactive iodine on an empty stomach. The iodine will be concentrated in the thyroid gland or excreted in the urine over the next few hours. The amount of iodine that is taken up by the thyroid gland is then measured to determine how well your thyroid functions.

Most of your iodine supply (70–80 percent) is located in your thyroid gland. However, there are iodine receptor sites located throughout your endocrine system and also in the breast, ovaries, and prostate. When these receptor sites are filled with dietary and supplemental iodine, your body becomes a shield from the lesser or toxic radioactive form of iodine from environmental toxic sources like the air and water contaminated from Fukushima. You *must* have enough dietary or supplemental iodine-filled receptor sites to shield your breast tissue, ovaries, and prostate gland from radiation.

Iodine is a halogen, like chlorine, fluorine, etc. and as such, can be absorbed through your skin. If you go out in the rain, and that rain carries radioactive iodine, it will be absorbed the minute it hits your skin and will be "taken up" by the thyroid. If you swim in ocean water contaminated by radioactive iodine, the same thing occurs, just like if you swim in a pool filled with chlorinated water. One theory to prevent this from happening is to *proactively* saturate yourself with iodine so you don't absorb the radioactive kind. If your thyroid receptor sites are full of beneficial iodine from dietary sources and supplements, they won't be able to absorb the harmful radioactive kind.

Supplemental iodine was very popular in the 1920s and '30s and was added to things like flour and salt to help correct deficiencies. But that is not the case anymore, and in fact, iodine intake has declined 50 percent in North America in the past thirty to forty years.

The consequences of this decline are dramatic as well. There have been epidemic increases in breast, thyroid, ovarian, prostate, and uterine cancers. The research relating iodine deficiency to breast cancer alone dates back more than one hundred years and is well documented and difficult to ignore. Even The World Health Organization cites iodine deficiency as "the most preventable cause of mental retardation" (Farrow, 2014). In addition, iodine was known to be effective against every pathogenic organism and listed in the Merck Manual as far back as 1899.

To see if you are iodine deficient, you can try a simple self-test at home. You can buy red-colored tincture of iodine at most drugstores. Put a little of it on a cotton swab or cotton ball and paint a small circle on your inner thigh or arm. If the yellow-orange stain is absorbed quickly and disappears within one to four hours, you may be iodine deficient. If the stain remains for four or more hours, you most likely have adequate amounts of iodine. This is just a preliminary test. Work with your doctor and a qualified laboratory for the most accurate results.

We must proactively saturate our iodine receptors daily with high-quality supplemental iodine to correct deficiencies, and we must minimize our exposure to external environmental radioactive sources that are competing for receptors. The sea vegetable kelp is a natural bioavailable form of iodine that comes in many dietary and supplement forms. Chlorophyll is another excellent way to purify and neutralize toxins. There are many iodine supplements as well and if you want to learn more, you should work with a knowledgeable health care professional to find what is best for you.

## RESOURCES:

All about Iodine
www.DrBrownstein.com

Farrow, L. *The Iodine Crisis.*
http://www.womentowomen.com/hypothyroidism/
iodinedeficiency-thyroidhealth.aspx

www.womentowomen.com/hypothyroidism/iodinedeficiency-
thyroidhealth.aspx

http://iodinehistory.blogspot.com/2012/08/merck-manual-1899.
html

chapter twenty

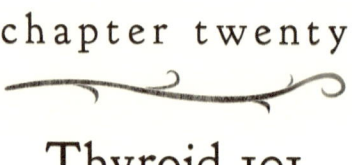

# Thyroid 101

The function of your thyroid gland is to take dietary or supplemental iodine from your bloodstream and make thyroid hormones. The names of the thyroid hormones reflect the number of iodine molecules attached—for example, T3 (triiodothyronine) has three iodine molecules attached, and T4 (thyroxine) has four. Thyroid hormones control heart rate, temperature, metabolism, glucose consumption, cortisol (stress hormone) regulation, and immune function.

As it is with all hormones, when looking at your body holistically, at the cellular level, disruption of one group of hormones *always* affects every other group of hormones. Your body is miraculously designed to *always* protect you, maintain homeostasis, and keep you alive. Your body *never* works against you. From a natural, holistic, cellular-level approach to healing, iodine is found in every single one of your hundred trillion cells. One could conclude then that the element iodine is essential to *life*.

This is not a new concept. Natural healers have known this since the beginning of time. Early studies in the 1900s proved that iodine *reversed* goiter. (Dr. David Marine gave iodine to two thousand schoolgirls over a 2 ½ year period with notable success—link below) This study was the reason the United States began to iodize salt. Supplemental iodine was added to bread—each slice contained about one hundred micrograms of iodine.

Then came the infamous "Wolff-Chaikoff" study (detailed previously), with questionable data stating iodine *caused* goiter in lab rats. Thus began the removal of iodine from bread and salt and the replacement of iodine with *bromine*. (See link below for more info.)

*Bromine is one of the most toxic, cancer-causing substances on the planet. Bromine forces iodine from your body by a process called competitive inhibition.*

So let's talk about the evil stepbrothers of iodine. Iodine is a member of the halogen family. Bromine, chlorine, and fluorine are all in competition for iodine receptors in your body. Iodine, in its elemental form, taken up by the thyroid and deposited in the many bodily receptors, is first used to *detoxify* your body of the other harmful halogens. However, you *must* have enough iodine initially to both support thyroid function, and fill those receptors. You must get the necessary elemental mineral salts in those endocrine-system receptor sites so you don't *absorb* the lower-quality halogens bromine, chlorine, fluoride, or radioactive iodine, which compete for receptor sites and force iodine out of the body, replacing the necessary mineral with the cancer causing toxins.

This is why the radioactive fallout from Chernobyl and Fukushima (previously stated) is so harmful. *Radiation from medical procedures is harmful as well.* Chlorinated water and fluoridated water is harmful. All of these halogens force iodine out of the body and fill receptor sites with toxic, cancer-causing substances. Perchlorate from rocket fuel, fireworks, flares, bleach, explosives, and fertilizer displaces iodine at a ratio of one perchlorate atom displacing one hundred iodine atoms. Ethylene dibromide from chemtrails forces out iodine as well.

According to Dr. Cousens, your skin holds four hundred milligrams of iodine, so you can understand why the halogens are so quickly absorbed by your body. The breasts, by the way, hold two hundred milligrams; the thyroid fifty milligrams.

Natural, elemental salts are *endothermic* and draw heat (a.k.a. inflammation) out of the body and combine with water to rehydrate the intestines, tissues, and glands. Radioactive substances burn internally, dehydrate, and cause oxidative stress and inflammation.

Bromine, *the most toxic, chemical, iodine-depleting substance in the world,* is such an insidious part of our environment that most people have no clue how much they are exposed to, and take in, on a daily basis.

Sources of bromine:

» Methyl bromide—a pesticide used on strawberries
» Potassium bromate—a dough conditioner found in commercial bakery products, some flours, and bread
» Brominated vegetable oil (BVO) —added to citrus drinks (Mountain Dew being the worst) and in red Gatorade
» Plastic parts used to make computers
» Medications—like Atrovent inhaler, nasal spray; Pro-Banthine, anesthesia
» Fire retardants used in infant and children pajamas, mattress pads, mattresses, carpets, upholstery
» Hot tub and pool cleaners
» In addition to bromine—fluoride in water and toothpaste. Ever wonder why you aren't supposed to swallow it? Fluorine is used in chemical warfare and dissolves bones and teeth.
» Triclosan—chemical found in antibacterial soap, body wash, toothpaste, cosmetics, toys, kitchen items

You have to feel sorry for iodine, don't you? Those are some *wicked* stepbrothers. Is it any wonder we are iodine deficient?

Iodine prevents and protects against breast and other cancers. When the body can't immediately eliminate toxins, it does one of two things. Incoming pathogens are surrounded by lymph tissue (like tonsils and adenoids), and internal toxins are stored in fat until they can be eliminated. Cancer-causing halogens are forced out of these tissues and glands by iodine sufficiency and saturation. Without enough iodine, the halogens deposit themselves and take up residence, causing inflammation, cysts, and cancer. Fluoride in particular accumulates in the thyroid and pineal glands. The pineal gland produces the hormones serotonin and melatonin. Fluoride interferes with the secretion of melatonin, causing calcium deposits in the pineal gland.

According to Dr. Gabriel Cousens, citing a study in the *International Journal of Radiation Biology*, Vol. 86, No. 12, December 2010, 1106–16, cordless phones, cell phones, and the "smart meters" used by utility companies with 900 MHz pulsed radiation cause hypothyroidism.

Radioactive isotopes from any source are a major problem. According to Dr. Cousens, Dr. Alice Stewart in 1955, studied women exposed to diagnostic X-rays during their pregnancies. She found that their babies were two times more likely to develop leukemia than babies who had not been exposed while in utero; and if the babies were exposed to X-rays in the first three months of pregnancy, they were twelve times more likely to develop childhood leukemia. If an infant is exposed to radioactive elements like strontium-90, the radioactive particles accumulate in the *bone marrow* and disrupt the developing immune system. Strontium-90 has a radioactive lifetime of 560 years—which means they continue to give off radiation for a long time as they decay. This causes damage on so many levels, even to the point of death.

In the eight months after the Chernobyl disaster, Massachusetts had the highest increase in infant mortality rates, with an increase of 900 percent for each thousand live births. This also happens in war-torn areas, where plutonium-239 was used. Again, these toxins remain in the soil forever—well— 500,000 years for plutonium. (This information is from *Conscious Eating* by Dr. Cousens, and my personal notes from naturopathy school.)

So how do we protect ourselves from radiation and the wicked stepbrothers of iodine? Let's all repeat my favorite mantra: "Pull out the poison, feed the body, and God will heal" (Burton Goldberg).

It goes without saying most of us are iodine deficient. To remedy that we need to supplement our iodine intake to make sure enough natural mineral-rich iodine is "taken up" to saturate the cells, tissues, and glands. By doing this, we prevent the lesser, toxic halogens from being absorbed and displacing iodine.

I choose kelp. I have been taking kelp supplements for years without any ill effects. You have to be careful with iodine supplements. There are many really good resources and qualified iodine specialists listed in *The Iodine Crisis* by Lynne Farrow, as well as websites and people to answer questions. Dr. Cousens and the Tree of Life Center have lots of resources as well. Start where you are. Find a doctor who will work with you.

Beets are a really great blood and liver detoxifier—specifically raw, organic beet juice. Beets are high in iron and have been successfully used for *years* to prevent and reverse radiation-caused cancers and leukemia. I make fresh apple-lemon-beet-wheatgrass juice in my juicer almost every day. I am a huge fan of fresh, organic juices. And I am blessed to call Jay Kordich, a.k.a. "The Juiceman," my mentor and friend. He is my juice expert and so knowledgeable about individual nutrients and juice combinations. You can read the chapter he wrote for me about juicing versus blending, or check out his Facebook page or website and ask him questions. I love people who are accessible to help share their knowledge, and I love people who radiate genuine kindness. Jay does both.

Switch to sea salt, or better yet, pink Himalayan salt. *Remember: your body needs the major minerals found in sea salt.* Elemental sodium (Na), potassium (K), and magnesium (Mg) are critical for cellular function. Sodium regulates your heartbeat. These salts combined with water *hydrate* your tissues and glands, providing moisture and lubrication. This is why with hypothyroidism you have dry skin, dry eyes, brittle nails, coarse hair. The halogen family members and radioactive iodine do the *opposite* —they burn you internally as they decompose, causing inflammation, dehydration, oxidative stress (fire rips through your oxygen stores), and eventual cell death.

Foods rich in chlorophyll protect against radiation, raise your pH, and build healthy red blood cells. Any green leafy foods will help (I like wheatgrass), but liquid chlorophyll is great too. I take Dr. Robert Young's pH Miracle Greens (Supergreens) every day.

One very effective strategy for "pulling out the poison" is called chelation. Chelation involves certain foods or products that actively draw radioactive toxins to them, bind them up, and eliminate them via the bowel, or in some cases, the skin. Sodium alginate sea vegetables, like my favorite, kelp, bind radioactive metals and prevent them from being absorbed in the body.

Protecting your thyroid and every other cell in your body can make such a difference in your quality of life, your protection against and recovery from cancer, and so many other chronic issues that I encourage you to use this information as a starting point. Don't take my word for it. The best research is that which is conducted with your own eyes in your own time.


## RESOURCES:

Link to Dr. David Marine study:
http://jn.nutrition.org/content/135/4/675.long

Dr. Alice Stewart Study 1955:
http://www.ratical.org/radiation/SecretFallout/SFchp2.html

Replacement of Iodine with Bromine:
http://beforeitsnews.com/health/2011/12/iodine-vs-bromine-what-they-are-not-telling-you-1467639.html

# Finding Your Truth and Living with Congruence: Is Your "Self-Talk" Killing You?

*I am by nature a dealer in words, and words are the*
*most powerful drug known to humanity.*
—Rudyard Kipling

One of the things people often ask me is, "If you could recommend one 'natural' thing for this (symptom, disease, condition), what would it be?" The truth is, there is no "one thing" that always works for that one thing. But there is *one thing* I know with absolute certainty after thirty years of studying, researching, and teaching healing:

## You Have to Find Your Personal Truth

Not my personal truth expressed here based on my experience; not your doctor's personal truth based on his; not truth based on statistics of people you don't know; not your sister's personal truth; not some movie star, rock star, or paid celebrity endorser's truth; and most importantly, not what you hear on TV.

People want a cure for cancer or diabetes, but they don't want to do what it requires of them to find that cure. Change is difficult. Healing requires introspection. They want to skip to the last chapter of the book without reading chapters one through all those that led up to it. We live in a world of instant gratification. We want to go from chapter 1 to 3 because chapter 3 holds what we perceive to be the answer. But first you have to answer the questions in chapter 2. Western medicine encourages this same "quick-fix" ideology. People want to take a pill to get rid of a symptom so they don't miss work, or taking the kids to soccer, or because they have a deadline, etc. People want to take a pill to treat their chest cold so they can continue smoking. It doesn't work that way. First you have to understand chapter 2. Chapter 2 explores the cause—it's like putting together the pieces of a puzzle to get to the source of your issue—and that takes time, and that starts in your mind.

There is no such thing as reality. There is only your perception of it. Your conscious mind is your filter. It decides how you perceive your world. Your subconscious mind is like an ATM or a computer. It can only respond to what you put in it or program it to do. The subconscious mind is power without direction—it has only one choice, and that is to obey. It listens to you speak and becomes a witness self or self-conscious. It carries out orders from your conscious mind without judgment or question.

Health is not obtained by constantly speaking of illness. Are you a cancer "victim"? That would depend on your perception. If you speak those words—cancer victim—your subconscious mind hears you. Victim implies you are a passive recipient of something outside your control. Victim implies fear. If you believe this as your truth, then you rely on outside forces to control your life. Fear is powerless. Fear is paralyzing and incapacitating.

Being a "victor" of cancer is also a choice. But that too depends on your perception. If you understand cancer grows inside you and therefore you have the power to change it, you become awakened, inspired, and empowered to take responsibility to heal, to choose to do something that *is* within your power. The same goes for any other illness or disease. Power is strength. Responsibility is not blame. Responsibility is putting the control back into your hands and telling yourself, "I can," "I'm capable," "I'm victorious."

## Words Matter

The subconscious mind is a habit mind. It learns by repetition. What you repeatedly and habitually tell yourself becomes your truth, despite outside appearances. That is why speaking words of love, health, and belief are so important. If you look at an anorexic person, you see a very thin unhealthy looking human being. But when an anorexic person looks in the mirror, she sees an unhealthy *fat* person. So despite *appearances* to the outside world, despite what might be considered reality—the perception when looking in the mirror is, "I'm fat."

People used to think affirmations were just "feel good, doesn't really have any effect on healing" type things. The study and research of psychoneuroimmunology has long since changed that outdated and incorrect truth. Mind imbalances or subconscious beliefs that we have been carrying around (sometimes outdated and downloaded from generations before us) have the most impact on the outcome of disease and longevity. If you believe cancer is going to kill you—it will. If you tell yourself, "I'd rather die than have to deal with my boss again tomorrow," you have a heart attack on Monday morning. Don't believe me? Look it up!

Psychoneuroimmunology teaches us that our thoughts transmit to neuropeptides (neuropeptides tell your immune system how to react and what hormones to release). Neuropeptides bind directly to immune cell surface receptors. Every immune cell has a receptor for a neuropeptide.

What you tell yourself repeatedly becomes your truth and forms conclusions. Conclusions then trigger your emotions and your emotions determine what hormones will be released. Are you stressed about failing a test? You release stress hormones. What you expect to happen becomes reality based on what you tell your subconscious to expect. Your body loves you and is always seeking balance. Therefore, the thoughts in your brain and the response of your immune system *must be congruent*. You can't have a negative thought or emotion in the brain without a corresponding negatively triggered hormonal or chemical release in your immune system. One chemical released by white blood cells, natural killer, and T-cells in response to an appropriate stimulus is *interferon*. Interferon is a naturally produced chemical that destroys cancer cells. If you can produce a substance that naturally kills cancer cells without the side effects of its synthetic counterpart—just by the words you emotionalize and repeatedly impress upon your subconscious mind—how important must those words be?

"Life and death are in the power of the tongue" (Proverbs 18:20).

One of my greatest teachers of the power of "self talk" is Louise Hay. She wrote an amazing book: *You Can Heal Your Life*.

I refer to her book with every client, friend, and loved one. The thoughts we repeatedly tell ourselves correspond to physical manifestations.

For most of my life, the person reflected in the mirror lived life from a place of fear. Fear of not being good enough, thin enough, worthy enough, smart enough, happy enough—fear of failing as a mother, wife, person—you get the picture. And those fears manifested as anger, depression, resentment, unforgiveness, competition, comparison.

All of which led to years of episodes of intense gallbladder pain. If you have ever experienced it, I don't need to tell you that it is unrelenting and incapacitating. If only I had known from the beginning that the root of my trouble wasn't *really* fatty food (although that was a contributor) but my unwillingness to forgive and my bitterness toward people who hurt me. Trust me when I say: A lesson is repeated until it is learned. Too late in my case; the stones were imbedded and my gallbladder removed.

The description in the book for "probable cause" of gallstones or "cholelithiasis" is "bitterness, hard thoughts, condemning, pride." The "new thought pattern" or affirmation is "there is joyous release of the past. Life is sweet, and so am I." While looking up a kidney issue for a client, I came upon another interesting realization. My mother died of Bright's Disease (a.k.a. acute or chronic nephritis). No one calls it that any more, so seeing it in Louise's book caught my eye. The probable cause: "Feeling like a kid who can't do it right and is not good enough. A failure. Loss." I guess that, along with my dad's legs and my grandmother's wild Italian spirit and cooking skills, my "DNA download" included some fears to address and work through. The affirmation or new thought pattern? "I love and approve of myself." And that's been the most difficult for me. The belief that "I'm worthy of being loved."

The reason I became a naturopathic doctor was because of the fear I saw in the eyes of people diagnosed with cancer. Western medicine feeds that fear. I have written about fear in many other chapters. Fear is paralyzing and incapacitating—not just in the case of cancer, but life in general. And that is where I was.

My role as a nurse and naturopathic doctor is to awaken, educate, and inspire you to find your own personal truth about what it means to you to live a vibrant healthy life, and to help you find the path to achieve it. Fear is paralyzing; knowledge is empowering.

## RESOURCES:

Hay, L. *You Can Heal Your Life.* (Louise and Hay House have many amazing books. All of Dr. Wayne Dyer's are my favorite too!) http://healyourlife.com.

Florence Scovel Shinn_wrote *The Game of Life and How to Play It,* which she published in 1925 herself. You can download it free. I have all of her books (The Complete Works) and I read them every day. http://florencescovelshinn.wwwhubs.com.

Here is one of my favorite Florence Scovel Shinn quotes: "We must substitute faith for fear, for fear is only inverted faith; it is faith in evil instead of good."

http://sacred-texts.com/nth/shinn/gol/index.htm (free copy of *The Game of Life and How to Play It*).

EVOX therapy uses your voice to reframe negative experiences in your life both past and present. It works to change your perception of emotional issues by reframing them in a positive way. http://www.zyto.com/evox.html.

# chapter twenty-two

## The Three Treasures—
## Share Your Light

If I had to choose one healing philosophy that truly resonates with me, it would be the ancient Daoist philosophy of the Three Treasures. In the last two years while writing this book, I have learned so much about this ancient, beautiful way of life, which is so congruent with everything I understand about true healing. Daoism is the fundamental Asian philosophy of living in balance and harmony with nature. The Three Treasures are the three energies the Chinese believe make up your entire life. The best way to begin to explain it is with the often-described analogy of the candle.

The first treasure is *jing*, meaning "essence," which is the accumulated life force of every one of your ancestors. It is the core of who you are physically, emotionally, and spiritually. Jing is your genetic blueprint and determines both vitality of life and life span.

At conception, the essence of mother and father become one within the new fetal cell. This united essence creates the energy that will sustain this new human being for life. This is "prenatal jing" or "original jing." Prenatal jing is what you inherit from your parents and determines how long you live, how much vitality, inner strength, and fortitude you bring to this life. After birth, original jing becomes actively involved in the process of converting food to energy. It is then considered postnatal jing, or simply jing. Jing is used up in the body by activities of daily living—but most especially by stress, excessive behaviors—and violating the natural laws of restful sleep, deep breathing, and conscious eating. Most westernized humans use up and "leak" jing as opposed to storing it.

The vitality of life is not measured in money, talent, or titles—it is our ability to *adapt* to the circumstances, opportunities, and stresses of our life. Jing is the root of our ability to adapt to every experience in our life. When jing runs low, we must tap into our original jing reserves—stored in each of our five primary organs (lungs, kidneys, liver, heart, and spleen). When you continually draw upon your original jing reserves, your life force is diminished, and you lose your ability to adapt. Your original jing, collectively inherited from all your ancestors all the way back to your Creator—contains within it every piece of information you need to know to adapt to your physical life on earth. You don't need to study—you just need to remember. Your life is a tapestry of all those who came before you. Everything your ancestors adapted to, overcame, and achieved is contained within your memory.

When original jing is depleted below a level required for survival, you die. "Leaking" jing is defined as loss of energy from any of the five organ storage sites. In order to promote longevity and preserve the physical body, a master practitioner of Chinese medicine must determine where energy is being leaked, why it is being leaked, stop the leak and restore energy to the particular organ and restore balance to the whole. The biggest leak of energy is chronic inflammation. *The Chinese have known for thousands of years that if you increase circulation and immunity, you will have increased vitality and longevity.* There are special tonics and practices that fortify jing. Ancient Chinese practitioners developed these in order to restore the leaked energy and build up large reserves of energy for future use. True health was considered "health beyond danger."

The second treasure in the Chinese Daoist system of medicine is *"qi (chi) or "vitality."* The word *qi* means "life force energy." In the Three Treasures system of healing arts, qi includes both energy and blood, and is believed to be the energy that animates us. Qi is both nourishing and protective. We build and restore qi every day by the food we eat and the air we breathe. *Ki* means the same in Japanese, and *Prana* in Hindi. Qi is the source of life that runs through every living being. This is the energy we tap into with tai chi and qigong and is the ki in Reiki. These three energy-restoring practices help us to replenish and store our jing energy instead of leaking it. Ancient TCM practitioners believed that the kidneys were the "gate of life." In Eastern philosophy, all disease can be traced to the kidneys. TCM practitioners always strengthen and regulate kidney function regardless of disease and even in the absence of any disorder.

Our kidneys are the "root" of our being and the place where jing is stored. Kidney jing is fluid like and forms the basis for growth, development, sexual maturation, and reproduction. Kidney jing produces "marrow" which in turn, produces bone marrow. When your red blood cells are not carrying oxygen throughout the river of life known as your bloodstream, and they are not picking up and removing acid wastes and gases, your body starts to acidify. As you begin storing acids and toxins and become oxygen deprived, your lungs must work harder to blow off carbon dioxide and you begin to hyperventilate. If you stimulate the kidneys through acupressure or qigong, they release a substance called *erythropoietin,* which stimulates your bone marrow to make more red blood cells. (Western medicine measures this by a blood test called a *reticulocyte count.*) At the ends of your femur and other bones you have a soft, spongy part called the epiphysis. As we age and make fewer healthy red blood cells, the quality of the marrow declines. When you stimulate the kidneys, the energy vitalizes the marrow to produce strong red blood cells, which in turn produce a stronger oxygen rich life force that flows throughout the entire body. You can restore energy and youthfulness over time by strengthening kidney function. This in turn balances erythropoietin (EPO) hormone function, which in turn balances bone marrow and therefore regulates red blood cell production. This builds new energy and increases red and white blood cell production in the marrow, which builds strong immunity.

This natural process of hormonal communication between erythropoietin in the kidneys and stem cells in the bone marrow to make more red blood cells when blood oxygen levels are low is preprogrammed in your body. Without your knowledge of how to strengthen and restore vital energy, your body, on its own, will begin to age and decompose because it is the cycle of life and the natural order of things. When your bone marrow dries up (due to dehydration), you won't produce the B cells, the NK cells, the T cells; your immune system grows weaker; good bacteria begin to lose the battle as bad bacteria seize the opportunity to develop strongholds throughout your intestines and bowel; your pH level starts to change as you lose the ability to eliminate these toxins; you acquire more packed acids and toxins; your internal terrain becomes more hospitable for bad bacteria to grow stronger and multiply and eventually take over your body, the host.

This is why the blood must be slightly alkaline and your immune system must have healthy bacteria and strong "marrow."

When you are filled with qi, you feel amazing—like you can do anything you chose to accomplish, you are confident, creative, happy and well balanced, filled with vital energy—fully alive yet peaceful. This is real *health*, as opposed to merely the absence of illness. The energy we use to heal our bodies and heal others comes from the kidney. Kidney health works closely with cardiovascular and heart health as well as giving us a strong will and nerves of steel that help us overcome the stresses of life.

Just like the root of a plant, the kidneys are the deepest source of life-giving energy to every human being. Sunlight energizes plants and empowers them to live, while their roots take in minerals and water for nourishment. Sunlight and water are essential to all life. Plants absorb the energy of sunlight and water and store it as chlorophyll. When we consume them, they enliven and empower us and build our blood. When we become enlivened, then we can offer our vital healing energy to those around us.

Think of a beautiful tree. A tree must first grow strong roots to absorb water and nutrients from the earth. Every day the tree opens its leaves and receives the energy and light from the sun. If the tree is deprived of water or cut down it dries out. Eventually, the tree will decompose and return to the earth. If we burn the tree as firewood—the stored energy will manifest as fire to give us heat and *light*.

Which brings us to the third treasure, *shen*.

Shen is spirit. The Daoists refer to it as "that which cannot be named." Some call it higher consciousness. Shen is the Divine love that is the core of our being and lives in the heart.

True Spirit allows each of us to be one with everything. Each of us possess this Universal, God-given Source of miraculous electromagnetic life force energy that flows through every cell of our body. Every living being, no matter what race, religion, culture, or belief system can attain this state of peaceful, higher conscious joy of *being*. Shen is the immortal or eternal aspect of our human being. The Daoists spent thousands of years cultivating the art form of tonic herbalism to extend life. They believed if they could extend their physical life, they could become more spiritual and develop their shen. The ultimate purpose of tonic herbalism was to nourish one or more of the three treasures and allow people more time to expand their Soul. It is necessary to nourish and protect both jing and qi so that shen has a physical "temple" to reside in and from which to radiate. This is why our body is our physical "temple" and must be cared for as the home of our sacred, eternal soul. All human disease is based on a lack of energy. Most of us are so busy "doing" that we don't take time to "be." So many things are competing for our attention and we are constantly being bombarded with electrical devices that steal our energy—computers, cell phones, TVs, etc. These things take us away from nature, peace, and stillness. We have lost our connection to nature. We look for some type of escape—pills to numb us, medication to take away our pain, and drinks to dull our fears—but you can't escape your way to a vibrant, purpose-driven life fulfilled. First you have to find your purpose. Get a dream.

Life is based on emotions. Are you happy and fulfilled, or are you stressed? Stress is another word for fear. Almost ninety percent of all doctor visits are caused by fear/stress. Everything you ever manifest on the outside was first created on the inside by the decisions you consciously make about what things mean, what to focus on, and what is important. Fear is a huge part of disease. Most people are afraid of things that will never happen. Fear is a powerful drain of vital energy. We are taught to hide our emotions of fear, disappointment, doubt, lack of self-love—but you must work through and master your mind and emotions. The role of genetics is not to worry about some future disease, but to reconnect with your ancestors. The emotional DNA that is downloaded from at least three generations is often times repeated unconsciously. Fear is the only emotion that separates you from your perfect self-expression or your true "essence." You must choose to live consciously every day and fill your mind with emotions of love—the most important being self-love.

So this is the process of aging. When you tell yourself your aches and pains are because "I'm getting old," your body listens. You begin to dehydrate and decay. Your body does what it is designed to do by natural order. Watch your "self-talk"!

Florence Scovel Shinn, one of my favorite authors, says this: "The imagination, the scissors of the mind, is constantly cutting out the events to come into your life. Many people are cutting out fear pictures. Seeing things that are not divinely planned. The seat of the imagining faculty is situated in the forehead [between the eyes]. Let the third eye be the watchman at the gate."

Florence is speaking of a tiny yet critically important gland that is located in your forehead right between your eyes. The ancients have called the *pineal gland,* "the third eye," "spirit valley," or the "seat of the soul." The pineal gland is a highly magnetic light receptor. Light is absorbed through the nerve endings of your retina, which act as a net to capture the light. Our body is lined up with the earth's energy or magnetism, otherwise known as circadian rhythm. Birds migrate on the basis of this intelligence and magnetism, and whales navigate the entire ocean using this gland. The pineal gland secretes the hormone *melatonin.* Melatonin is the hormone of darkness and its release is dependent upon a balance of light and dark cycles. Melatonin is important for keeping your body in balance with circadian rhythm—telling it whether it is night or day—winter or summer. Disruptions in nighttime melatonin levels produce adverse affects. Dr. Steven Lockley of Brigham and Women's Hospital, Harvard University is studying the role this disruption plays in cancer and bone loss. Dr. Lockley is studying the impact of lack of light on bone rhythms of blind women and hopes to explain the loss of bone that occurs in night-shift workers.

In Western civilizations, the process of premature aging is happening to increasing numbers of young people. How many young men and women have cardiovascular disease? Cancer has touched almost every family. If your immune system is weak from years of suppressing acute infections with antibiotics and painkillers, then you have built systemic infection into your body, adding to years of chemically processed food, lack of sleep, no exercise, artificial light, poor water, dehydration—at this point your body is not much use to you, your species, or the earth. Bacteria do what they are designed to do by natural order. They break down **matter** and return it to the earth. You see, bacteria are not concerned with who you are, what you own, how young or old you are—bacteria know their life purpose and that is to break down matter and return the original elements to the earth to replenish the soil. Without the humble creatures of the earth breaking down our bodies into reusable elements, our planet would be covered with dead matter and new life would not be sustainable.

I think we are finally beginning to realize that we can't eat, drink, drug, or numb our way to an inspired, purpose-driven life.

You are here at this moment in time for a reason. You carry inside you all the experiences, knowledge, and wisdom of the ancients. My wish for you is that my truth, expressed here in this book, awakens, educates, empowers, and inspires you to expand your idea of true health or as the ancients would say, "health beyond danger." The only way to a vibrant, purpose-driven life—an extraordinary life—is to first decide what that means to you.

Brendon Burchard says in his new book, *The Charge,* "We are now a culture flooded with tasks and spreadsheets and work plans that inspire no heart, no drive, no courage. I say, you want to change? Then do not, under any circumstances, allow yourself to settle on a vision or a calling or a change in any arena that is uninspiring. If you're going to have clarity on something in your life, make it something so big and bright and meaningful that you will get out of bed and chase it until you grasp it or die."

The traditional analogy to begin to explain the philosophy of The Three Treasures is that of a candle.

The wax and the wick are finite and represent the essence, or jing. The size of the candle and length of the wick help determine the life expectancy of it. Jing represents both heredity and lifestyle. A conscious lifestyle in harmony with nature can extend the length of time the candle burns.

The flame of the candle is the energy manifested to provide the source of light. The flame eventually consumes the candle—burning slowly or rapidly—depending on the amount of energy. This is analogous to qi.

The ultimate purpose of the candle is to give *light.* The light given off by the candle is analogous to Shen. Shen is the Divine guiding light that lives in the heart of every human being. If all of us could come from our original *essence*—as opposed to our *fears*—in our daily activity, in all our interactions, communications, in all of our being—then each of us would be the light for one another.

May your heart and your light guide you to radiant health and a life fulfilled.

## RESOURCES:

*The Ancient Wisdom of the Chinese Tonic Herbs* by Ron Teeguarden. This man and this book will give you so much information about tonic herbs for specific conditions. The Three Treasures are so much more than you can write about in one chapter—the book and Ron's website are the best resource!

*The Secret Door to Success* by Florence Scovel Shinn--free PDF online: http://www.consciouslivingfoundation.org/ebooks/14-withcover/ CLF-The%20Secret%20Door%20To%20Success%20-%20 excerpts%20-%20Florence%20Scovel%20Shin.pdf

*Cultured Food for Life*—favorite author, book, and website for information on fermenting and putting good bacteria in your gut: http://www.culturedfoodlife.com/

My favorite "longevity sage"—Peter Ragnar has taught me so much. I love this qigong program! I love everything Peter teaches! http://www.longevitysage.com/filled-with-chi

Burchard, B. *The Charge:*
http://brendonburchard.com/

Sleep research study of blind women:
http://www.huffingtonpost.com/steven-lockley-phd

Ron Teeguarden's website with amazing information on herbal supplements and the research behind them:
www.dragonherbs.com

Erythropoietin test information:
http://www.nlm.nih.gov/medlineplus/ency/article/003683.htm

# About the Author

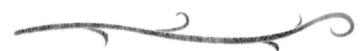

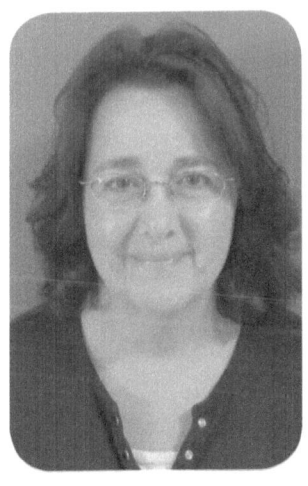

Thomasina (Tammy) Copenhaver, RN, BSN, ND is a registered nurse and naturopathic doctor with more than thirty years' experience in the health care profession. She started out as a candy striper and nurses' aide at King's Daughter's Hospital in Martinsburg, West Virginia. It was there that she decided to pursue a career in nursing. She completed her bachelor of science degree in nursing at West Virginia University and is a proud Mountaineer fan!

Following graduation, she worked in various clinical settings beginning with a community hospital, where she worked in every department in preparation for her nursing board exam. She left after two years to become a staff nurse at the Veteran's Administration hospital where she worked in the nursing home care unit. There she found her favorite group of people to work with and care for—the elderly. When her husband returned to college, she moved back to WVU and became assistant director of nursing at Sundale Nursing Home.

When her husband graduated, she moved again and taught nursing skills at Hagerstown Community College and worked for an orthopedic surgeon as his office and clinical nurse, and personal assistant. After her children were born she worked part time as a legal nurse consultant, advocating for nursing home abuse victims and workers' compensation rights.

After her husband was diagnosed with cancer and healed with surgery and natural methods, Tammy went to graduate school to become a doctor of naturopathy. For the last twelve years she has consulted with clients individually, free of charge, through word of mouth, friend to friend, educating them, juicing with them, sharing products at her kitchen table, and empowering them to take responsibility for their health through "conscious living." Through her blog and writing for both Examiner.com and NaturalNews. com/ blogs; she has helped people from as far away as Turkey and Fukushima, Japan.